I0841504

Gastric sleeve
versus
Gastric bypass

Bariatrics Unveiled: A Comprehensive
Guide to Weight Loss Surgery – Making the
Right Decision with Roux-en-Y Gastric
Bypass and Sleeve Gastrectomy

By Sara C. Blackmon

Copyright

© 2023 [Sara C. Blackmon]

Disclaimer

This book is intended for informational purposes only and is not a substitute for professional medical advice, diagnosis, or treatment. The author and publisher disclaim any liability or responsibility for any adverse consequences resulting directly or indirectly from the use of information presented in this book. Readers are encouraged to consult with qualified healthcare professionals for personalized medical guidance tailored to their individual circumstances.

The views and opinions expressed in this book are those of the author and do not necessarily reflect the official policy or position of any healthcare institution or organization. The author and publisher make no representations or warranties with respect to the accuracy, applicability, fitness, or completeness of the contents of this book. The inclusion of specific surgical procedures and medical information does not imply endorsement or guarantee of outcomes.

Every effort has been made to ensure that the information in this book is accurate at the time of publication. However, medical knowledge is constantly evolving, and new research may impact the understanding and recommendations provided. The author and publisher are not responsible for any errors or omissions or for the results obtained from the use of this information.

Gastric sleeve versus Gastric bypass *by Sara C. Blackmon*

About The Author

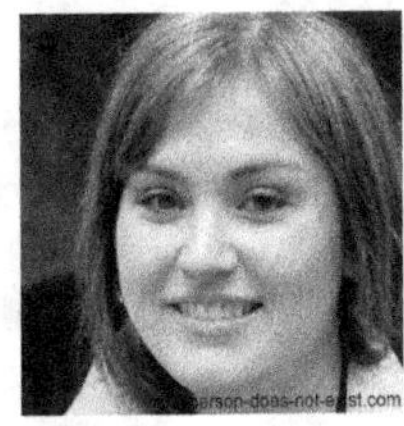

Dr. Sara C. Blackmon is a distinguished psychologist, author, and advocate for holistic well-being, with a profound commitment to guiding individuals on their transformative journeys. Holding a Ph.D. in Psychology, Sara combines her clinical expertise with a passion for empowering individuals to achieve optimal mental and physical health.

As a seasoned psychologist, Sara has dedicated her career to understanding the intricate connections between mental and physical wellness. Her extensive experience in clinical practice has uniquely positioned her to address the psychological aspects of weight loss surgery with empathy and insight.

Beyond her role as a psychologist, Sara is an accomplished author, weaving together her professional knowledge and personal understanding to create a bridge between the complexities of bariatric surgery and the emotional landscapes of those undergoing such transformative experiences. Her writing is characterized by a unique blend of clinical precision and compassionate storytelling.

Sara's commitment to the well-being of others is evident in her holistic approach to health. Her book not only explores the technicalities of weight loss surgery but delves deep into the emotional and psychological dimensions that shape the journey to a healthier and more fulfilling life.

Recognized for her ability to make complex psychological concepts accessible, Sara C. Blackmon seeks to empower readers with knowledge and resilience. Through her writing, she aims to dismantle stigma surrounding obesity and mental health, fostering a supportive and understanding community.

Table of content

Copyright/Disclaimer

The information contained in this book is for general instructional purposes only While the author has made every effort to provide accurate and up-to-date information, readers are advised to consult with relevant professionals, such as lawyers, therapists, or counselors, to address their specific concerns and needs related to the topics discussed in this book. The author and publisher shall not be liable for any negative consequences, harm, or legal consequences that may arise from the use or misuse of this book's contents.

While the author has made efforts to protect the privacy and confidentiality of individuals mentioned in the book, characters, and incidents are used for illustrative purposes and any resemblance to actual persons, living or dead, or actual scenario is completely coincidental.

Every effort has been made to respect the intellectual property rights of third parties, and the author and publisher will promptly address any verified claims of copyright infringement regarding materials used in the book, provided the necessary permission was not obtained.

Introduction

In a world where the battle of the bulge has become an all-too-common struggle, where the scale seems to tip further against our favor with each passing day, the quest for a healthier, happier life often begins with a challenging question: "How can I lose weight, and keep it off?"

Obesity, a global epidemic of our times, is not just about vanity or fitting into smaller-sized clothes. It's a complex issue with far-reaching implications for health, self-esteem, and overall well-being. For many, the journey to achieving and maintaining a healthy weight is filled with obstacles, plateaus, and moments of frustration. In the face of such challenges, weight loss surgery becomes a consideration.

This book, "Gastric Sleeve versus Gastric Bypass: A Comprehensive Guide to Weight Loss Surgery," is your essential companion in navigating this significant decision. Whether you are personally contemplating these surgical options, supporting a loved one in their journey, or simply seeking to understand the profound impact of weight loss surgery, you've come to the right place.

The purpose of this book is twofold: to empower you with the knowledge needed to make an informed choice and to provide a holistic understanding of the gastric sleeve and gastric bypass surgeries. We aim to shed light on the benefits, potential risks, and outcomes associated with these procedures. In doing so, we will help you uncover the path that aligns best with your unique circumstances, weight loss goals, and health needs.

As the author, I bring a deep commitment to this subject, grounded in a sincere desire to assist those facing the obesity challenge. My personal motivations stem from a genuine concern for the well-being of individuals who find themselves in the midst of the weight loss journey. Throughout this book, we'll explore the medical aspects, psychological aspects, and personal stories that shape the world of weight loss surgery. We'll provide you with a comprehensive guide so you can embark on your weight loss journey armed with knowledge, confidence, and a clear understanding of the choices before you.

Weight loss surgery is not a decision to be taken lightly, but it can be life-changing for those who are well-informed and prepared. As we delve into the pages ahead, you'll discover insights from healthcare professionals, real-life accounts from individuals who have undergone these procedures, and a wealth of practical advice to support your journey.

So, let's embark on this journey together. It's a journey toward a healthier, happier you, one in which knowledge, determination, and the right medical guidance can pave the way for transformative change. Welcome to "Gastric Sleeve versus Gastric Bypass: A Comprehensive Guide to Weight Loss Surgery." It's time to take the first step on the path to a healthier and more fulfilling life.

Understanding the Obesity Epidemic

Globally, the prevalence of overweight and obesity poses a serious threat to the prevention of chronic diseases and to people's health throughout their lives. Due to factors such as economic expansion, industrialization, mechanized transportation, urbanization, a shift toward processed foods and high-calorie diets, and an increasingly sedentary lifestyle, the prevalence of obesity in many countries has doubled or even tripled in the last 30 years. Particularly, the alarmingly high incidence of childhood obesity portends a devastating cost of disease for both individuals and healthcare systems in the years to come. Obesity is a multifaceted and intricate illness that has roots in genetics, behavior, socioeconomics, and the environment. It increases the risk of severe morbidity and mortality. This non-exhaustive study, which mostly relies on epidemiologic data released in the past 10 years, addresses the scope of the obesity pandemic, its known and unknown risk factors, consequences, and global economic impact.

Obesity, a global health crisis of epic proportions, is the starting point of our journey toward understanding the world of weight loss surgery. We'll delve into the various dimensions of the obesity epidemic, exploring its implications, and the factors that have driven it to the forefront of public health concerns.

Health Implications of Obesity

Obesity is not just a matter of aesthetics; it has far-reaching health implications. In this section, we'll uncover the myriad health risks associated with obesity, including cardiovascular diseases, diabetes, sleep apnea, joint problems, and mental health challenges. By comprehending the health consequences of obesity, you will gain a deeper insight into why weight loss is not merely a cosmetic endeavor but a life-saving one.

Factors Contributing to the Obesity Epidemic

The obesity epidemic did not happen overnight; it is the result of a complex interplay of factors. We will explore the societal, environmental, genetic, and behavioral factors contributing to the rise in obesity rates. Factors like sedentary lifestyles, poor dietary choices, and the obesogenic environment will be dissected to provide a comprehensive view of the forces at play.

Weight Loss Surgery as an Option

As we wrap up this section, we'll introduce the concept of weight loss surgery as a potential solution for individuals grappling with severe obesity. We'll discuss the origins of these surgical procedures and their role in addressing the obesity epidemic. The chapter will lay the foundation for the deeper exploration of gastric sleeve and gastric bypass surgeries, providing the context for the decision-making process ahead.

As we further, you will have a clearer understanding of the obesity epidemic, the urgent need for effective interventions, and the potential role of weight loss surgery as a powerful tool in the fight against obesity. This knowledge will serve as a solid foundation for the subsequent chapters, where we will dive deeper into the world of these surgical procedures.

Purpose and Scope of the Book

In your journey through the pages of "Gastric Sleeve versus Gastric Bypass: A Comprehensive Guide to Weight Loss Surgery," it is crucial to understand the precise intentions and the boundaries that frame this book.

Purpose:

The primary purpose of this book is to empower individuals who are considering weight loss surgery, those supporting loved ones in their weight loss journey, or anyone seeking comprehensive knowledge on the topic. Our aim is to provide you with a valuable resource that can guide you through the intricate world of gastric sleeve and gastric bypass surgeries. We want to help you make informed decisions by offering in-depth insights into the benefits, potential risks, outcomes, and considerations associated with these procedures.

Scope:

This book is not intended to replace professional medical advice. It does not offer personal medical recommendations or specific surgical advice. Rather, it serves as a bridge between you and healthcare professionals, equipping you with the knowledge needed to engage in meaningful discussions with your medical team.

The scope of this book encompasses the following areas:

- An exploration of the obesity epidemic, its definitions, and the health implications it carries.
- A detailed examination of gastric sleeve and gastric bypass surgeries, including their procedures, benefits, potential risks, and outcomes.
- A focus on the factors to consider when deciding which surgery aligns best with your weight loss goals, medical history, and lifestyle.
- Guidance on the pre-operative process, preparation for surgery, and addressing common concerns.
- An account of the surgical experience, what to expect on the day of surgery, and the role of the healthcare team.

- Insights into the recovery period and post-operative life, including dietary and lifestyle adjustments.
- A discussion on the long-term outcomes and potential complications associated with these surgical options.
- Guidance on aftercare, ongoing medical follow-ups, support groups, and maintaining a healthy lifestyle.
- Real-life stories and testimonials from individuals who have undergone these surgeries to provide personal insights.

The book will not delve into technical medical procedures, as it is not a manual for surgeons. Instead, it serves as a comprehensive guide for those seeking to understand the world of weight loss surgery from a patient's perspective.

The information contained within this book is current as of the knowledge cutoff date in January 2022. Medical practices and research may evolve over time, so it is essential to consult with your healthcare professionals for the most up-to-date information and personalized guidance.

Personal Motivations for Writing

Behind every book, especially one dealing with the profound subject of weight loss surgery, there are often deeply personal motivations that fuel the author's dedication to the topic. In this section, I'd like to share with you the driving forces behind the creation of "Gastric Sleeve versus Gastric Bypass: A Comprehensive Guide to Weight Loss Surgery."

A Compassion for Those on the Weight Loss Journey

At the core of my motivation lies a deep and abiding compassion for individuals who find themselves on the weight loss journey, particularly those who have been contending with the formidable challenge of obesity.

I've witnessed the physical and emotional toll that obesity can exact on individuals and their families, and it has fueled a desire to contribute positively to their well-being.

The Desire for Informed Decision-Making

I believe that every person, when faced with a decision as monumental as weight loss surgery, should have access to accurate, unbiased, and comprehensive information. Making an informed choice about one's health is a fundamental right, and my goal is to ensure that you, the reader, have the tools and insights needed to make choices that are in line with your particular goals and situation.

Demystifying the Complexities of Weight Loss Surgery

Weight loss surgery can seem shrouded in mystery, with medical jargon and technical details that may appear inscrutable to the layperson. My motivation is to demystify these complexities, to break down the barriers between medical terminology and plain language, so that anyone can understand the procedures, benefits, and potential risks involved in weight loss surgery.

Giving a Voice to Real-Life Experiences

In writing this book, I wanted to give voice to the real-life experiences of individuals who have undergone weight loss surgery. Their journeys, struggles, triumphs, and challenges are an integral part of the story. By sharing these personal narratives, my hope is that you can glean insights and inspiration from those who have walked this path before you.

Promoting Holistic Well-Being

Beyond the physical aspects of weight loss, I am motivated by a commitment to holistic well-being. This encompasses not only the physical health of individuals but also their emotional and psychological well-being. Weight loss surgery is not just about shedding pounds; it's about reclaiming one's life and happiness, and I am motivated to support that journey.

Understanding Obesity

Obesity, a pervasive health issue of our time, transcends mere numbers on a scale. It is a complex, multifaceted condition with significant implications for individual health, society, and healthcare systems worldwide. In this chapter, we will embark on a journey to gain a deeper understanding of obesity—what it is, why it matters, and how it impacts the lives of millions.

Defining Obesity

Defining obesity goes beyond mere numbers on a scale; it is a multifaceted health condition with profound implications for an individual's well-being. In this section, we will explore the various ways in which obesity is defined, diagnosed, and understood in the medical and public health contexts.

Body Mass Index (BMI)

One of the most common methods for defining obesity is through the calculation of Body Mass Index (BMI). BMI is a numeric value derived from a person's height and weight and is used to categorize individuals into different weight categories. These categories typically include:

Underweight: BMI less than 18.5
Normal weight: BMI 18.5 to 24.9
Overweight: BMI 25 to 29.9
Obesity (Class I): BMI 30 to 34.9
Obesity (Class II): BMI 35 to 39.9
Severe Obesity (Class III): BMI 40 or greater
While BMI is a valuable tool for quickly assessing weight status, it has limitations. It does not take into account variations in body composition or distinguish between muscle and fat mass. Therefore, it may not always provide an accurate reflection of an individual's health or risk factors.

Waist Circumference

In addition to BMI, waist circumference is another measure used to assess abdominal obesity. Excess fat around the abdomen, often referred to as visceral fat, is associated with a higher risk of obesity-related health conditions. Waist circumference measurements can provide additional information about a person's health status.

Body Composition

Body composition analysis, which considers the distribution of muscle and fat in the body, offers a more comprehensive view of an individual's health. It can help differentiate between lean body mass and fat mass, shedding light on the specific health risks associated with excess fat.

Diagnostic Criteria

To diagnose obesity, healthcare professionals often rely on a combination of factors, including BMI, waist circumference, and medical history. In clinical settings, physicians take into account an individual's overall health, lifestyle, and potential obesity-related health conditions to make a comprehensive assessment.

Understanding Obesity as a Health Condition

It's important to recognize that obesity is not solely about body weight; it is a complex health condition associated with numerous risk factors. These risk factors extend beyond physical health to encompass mental and emotional well-being, self-esteem, and overall quality of life. The consequences of obesity may include a higher risk of heart disease, type 2 diabetes, sleep apnea, certain cancers, and musculoskeletal problems, among others.

Health Implications of Obesity

Obesity, far from being a superficial concern, carries profound and far-reaching health implications. Let's delve into the extensive health consequences associated with obesity, emphasizing the critical need to address this condition not just for cosmetic reasons but to safeguard one's overall well-being.

Cardiovascular Diseases

One important risk factor for cardiovascular illnesses is obesity. Excess body fat can lead to conditions like high blood pressure (hypertension), atherosclerosis (narrowing of the arteries), and an increased risk of heart disease. The cardiovascular system is strained because the heart must work harder to pump blood.

Type 2 Diabetes

There is a strong correlation between type 2 diabetes and obesity. Excess fat, especially around the abdomen, can disrupt the body's ability to regulate blood sugar. Over time, this can lead to insulin resistance, where the body's cells do not respond effectively to insulin, resulting in elevated blood sugar levels.

Sleep Apnea

Obesity is a leading cause of obstructive sleep apnea, a condition where breathing repeatedly stops and starts during sleep. This can lead to disrupted sleep patterns, daytime fatigue, and an increased risk of other health issues such as cardiovascular disease.

Certain Cancers

Obesity is associated with an increased risk of several types of cancer, including breast, colon, and endometrial cancers. The exact mechanisms behind this link are still under investigation, but it may be related to hormonal changes and inflammation associated with excess body fat.

Joint Problems

Excess weight puts additional stress on the joints, particularly the knees, hips, and lower back. This can lead to conditions such as osteoarthritis, causing pain, reduced mobility, and a diminished quality of life.

Mental Health Challenges

Obesity often leads to emotional and psychological challenges. Individuals with obesity may experience lower self-esteem, body image issues, and depression. Social stigmas and discrimination can compound these challenges, leading to further mental health issues.

Quality of Life

An individual's overall quality of life can be considerably diminished by obesity. Day-to-day activities may become more challenging, leading to a diminished sense of well-being and vitality. The physical and emotional toll of obesity can impact relationships, work, and overall life satisfaction.

Reproductive Health

Obesity can affect reproductive health, leading to fertility issues in both men and women. In women, it can disrupt menstrual cycles and lead to complications during pregnancy. It may exacerbate erectile dysfunction in men.

Respiratory Problems

Obesity is associated with an increased risk of respiratory problems such as asthma and reduced lung function. The excess fat can restrict the movement of the diaphragm and chest wall, making it harder to breathe.

Factors Contributing to the Obesity Epidemic

The obesity epidemic is not the result of a single cause but rather a complex interplay of various factors. Understanding these contributing factors is essential in addressing and combating the rising rates of obesity worldwide. Here, we will explore the multifaceted elements that have led to the obesity epidemic.

Sedentary Lifestyles

Modern technology and changes in the nature of work have led to increasingly sedentary lifestyles. Many people spend more time sitting at desks, watching screens, or using motorized transportation, which reduces physical activity and contributes to weight gain.

Poor Dietary Choices

Highly processed, calorie-dense, and nutrient-poor foods have become more accessible and prevalent. Fast food, sugary drinks, and snack foods often dominate diets, displacing healthier, whole foods. This shift in dietary patterns can lead to weight gain and obesity.

Environmental Factors

The environment in which people live plays a significant role in obesity rates. Factors such as food availability, accessibility, and advertising can influence dietary choices. Additionally, "food deserts," areas with limited access to affordable, healthy foods, can contribute to poor eating habits.

Marketing and Advertising

The food industry often heavily markets and advertises unhealthy products, particularly to children. This can lead to the consumption of high-calorie, low-nutrient foods and beverages.

Genetics

Genetics can influence a person's propensity to become obese. Some people may have a genetic predisposition that makes it easier for them to gain weight or have difficulty losing it. However, genetics alone do not determine obesity; environmental and lifestyle factors also play a crucial role.

Socioeconomic Factors

Low socioeconomic status is often associated with higher obesity rates. Limited financial resources can make it more challenging to access healthy foods, engage in physical activity, or afford healthcare, which can contribute to weight gain.

Stress and Emotional Factors

Stress, anxiety, and emotional factors can lead to overeating or unhealthy eating habits as a coping mechanism. Emotional eating can be a significant contributor to obesity.

Lack of Physical Education

Reduced emphasis on physical education in schools and decreased opportunities for physical activity can limit children's exposure to healthy behaviors and contribute to obesity.

Urban Design

Urban environment design has an impact on physical activity. Communities that lack safe, walkable spaces, parks, and recreational facilities may discourage physical activity.

Cultural and Social Norms

Cultural and social norms can affect eating habits and body image. In some cultures, larger body sizes may be viewed as attractive, while in others, there may be pressure to conform to specific body ideals.

Weight Loss Surgery as an Option

Weight loss surgery, also known as bariatric surgery, is a medical intervention that has gained prominence as an effective and potentially life-changing option for individuals struggling with severe obesity. Here we would discuss the world of weight loss surgery, exploring its history, the various surgical procedures, and the considerations that make it a viable choice for those on their journey to better health.

A Historical Perspective

Weight loss surgery has a rich history dating back decades. The first successful weight loss surgery, known as jejunoileal bypass, was performed in the 1950s, at the University of Minnesota . However, it was associated with numerous complications and fell out of favor. Over time, surgical techniques evolved, leading to the development of safer and more effective procedures. Today, bariatric surgery has become a well-established and increasingly refined field of medicine.

The Role of Weight Loss Surgery

Weight loss surgery is not a cosmetic procedure; it is a medical intervention aimed at addressing severe obesity and its associated health risks. Its primary goals are to achieve significant weight loss, improve or resolve obesity-related health conditions, and enhance an individual's overall quality of life.

Considerations for Weight Loss Surgery

Weight loss surgery is a major decision and not suitable for everyone. Prior to following this course, it is crucial to take into account the following factors:

Weight and Health Status: Weight loss surgery is typically recommended for individuals with a BMI of 40 or higher, or a BMI of 35-39.9 with significant obesity-related health conditions.

Medical Evaluation: Thorough medical evaluations are conducted to assess a person's overall health and readiness for surgery.

Commitment to Lifestyle Changes: Weight loss surgery is most effective when combined with lifelong changes in diet, exercise, and behavior.

Support System: Having a supportive network of friends and family can be invaluable during the weight loss journey.

Realistic Expectations: It's essential to have realistic expectations about the outcomes of weight loss surgery.

Potential Risks and Complications: Like any surgical procedure, weight loss surgery carries certain risks and potential complications that need to be understood.

Overview of Weight Loss Surgery

Weight loss surgery, also known as bariatric surgery, has emerged as a powerful and effective tool for individuals battling severe obesity. In this chapter, we'll provide an in-depth overview of weight loss surgery, covering the different types of procedures, the principles underlying their success, and the crucial role of healthcare professionals in guiding patients through this transformative journey.

Types of Weight Loss Surgery

Several weight loss surgical procedures are available, each with its own advantages and considerations. The two major categories of weight loss surgeries are restrictive procedures and malabsorptive procedures. The most common surgical options include:

Gastric Sleeve (Sleeve Gastrectomy): This procedure involves removing a portion of the stomach, reducing its size and capacity. It restricts the amount of food an individual can consume, leading to early satiety and weight loss.

Gastric Bypass (Roux-en-Y): Gastric bypass combines restriction and malabsorption. It creates a small stomach pouch and re-routes the small intestine to limit calorie absorption. This procedure results in both reduced food intake and decreased calorie absorption.

Lap-Band (Adjustable Gastric Banding): A restrictive procedure, the Lap-Band involves placing an adjustable band around the upper part of the stomach. It can be tightened or loosened to control food intake.

Biliopancreatic Diversion with Duodenal Switch (BPD/DS): This is a malabsorptive and restrictive procedure that involves reducing stomach size and rerouting the small intestine. It results in significant weight loss and decreased calorie absorption.

The Role of Healthcare Professionals

Weight loss surgery is a significant medical intervention that requires careful evaluation, expert guidance, and ongoing support to ensure its success. In this chapter, we will explore the essential role of healthcare professionals in every stage of the weight loss surgery journey, from initial evaluation to long-term aftercare.

1. Preoperative Evaluation

Before individuals undergo weight loss surgery, they undergo a comprehensive preoperative evaluation conducted by a team of healthcare professionals, including:

Bariatric Surgeon: The surgeon specializes in performing weight loss surgeries. They assess a patient's overall health, determine surgical eligibility, and explain the procedure's risks and benefits.

Dietitian: Dietitians provide nutritional counseling and guidance. They help individuals prepare for surgery by teaching them how to follow a pre-surgery diet and explaining post-surgery dietary requirements.

Psychologist or Psychiatrist: Mental health professionals evaluate a patient's psychological readiness for surgery. They assess the patient's understanding of the emotional and lifestyle changes that accompany weight loss surgery.

Internal Medicine or Primary Care Physician: The patient's primary care physician plays a crucial role in ensuring that they are in optimal health for surgery. They may manage and optimize pre-existing medical conditions.

2. Surgical Procedure

During the surgery itself, the bariatric surgeon is the central healthcare professional responsible for performing the weight loss surgery. The surgery may involve complex techniques, depending on the chosen procedure. The surgeon works with an operating room team to ensure the procedure is carried out safely and effectively.

3. Post-operative Care

After surgery, individuals receive care and support from a multidisciplinary team of healthcare professionals to promote a successful recovery and long-term success. This team may include:

Dietitian: Post-surgery, dietitians continue to provide guidance on dietary changes and supplementation to ensure proper nutrition.

Nurse or Nurse Practitioner: Nurses monitor patients for any immediate post-surgery complications and provide education on wound care, pain management, and any red flags to watch for.

Psychologist or Counselor: Ongoing psychological support helps individuals navigate the emotional and mental aspects of the post-surgery journey. It addresses issues like body image, emotional eating, and adjustment to lifestyle changes.

Exercise Specialist or Physical Therapist: Professionals in this category help patients develop appropriate exercise plans to maintain or increase physical activity levels, improving overall fitness.

Support Groups: Many bariatric surgery programs offer support groups where individuals can connect with peers who have gone through similar experiences, providing a valuable network of emotional support.

4. Long-term Follow-up

The role of healthcare professionals doesn't end with the surgery and immediate post-operative care. Long-term follow-up and support are crucial for maintaining weight loss and addressing any potential complications or issues. The follow-up team may include:

- **Bariatric Surgeon:** The surgeon continues to monitor the patient's health and assess any potential complications or issues related to the surgical procedure.

- **Dietitian**: Dietitians provide ongoing guidance on nutrition, portion control, and long-term dietary choices to ensure continued success.

- **Psychologist or Counselor:** Psychological support remains vital to address any emotional challenges or psychological factors that may impact weight loss and overall well-being.

- **Primary Care Physician:** The patient's primary care physician continues to manage general health, monitor pre-existing medical conditions, and coordinate care with the bariatric team.

- **Endocrinologist:** If the patient has diabetes, an endocrinologist may manage and adjust medications as weight loss progresses.

- **Physical Therapist or Exercise Specialist:** Exercise professionals support patients in maintaining physical activity and fitness, adapting exercise plans as needed.

Gastric Sleeve Surgery

Gastric sleeve surgery, also known as sleeve gastrectomy, is a highly effective and increasingly popular weight loss surgery that has transformed the lives of countless individuals struggling with obesity. In this chapter, we will provide a comprehensive overview of gastric sleeve surgery, including its procedure, benefits, potential risks, and what individuals can expect when choosing this path to better health.

Procedure:

Gastric sleeve surgery involves the surgical reduction of the stomach's size, leading to a restriction in food intake. This is a detailed breakdown of the process:

Stomach Reshaping: The surgeon begins by making several small incisions in the abdomen. Through these incisions, they access the stomach.

Stapling and Resection: The next step involves the use of a stapling device to divide the stomach into two sections. The larger portion, which makes up the majority of the stomach, is removed, leaving behind a small, banana-shaped stomach or "sleeve."

Suture Closure: The surgeon then uses sutures to close and seal the newly created stomach pouch.

Surgical Finish: The removed portion of the stomach is excised from the body.

Benefits of Gastric Sleeve

Significant Weight Loss: Gastric sleeve surgery is renowned for its ability to promote substantial and sustainable weight loss. Many patients experience significant reductions in their excess body weight, often ranging from 50% to 80% within the first year following surgery. This weight loss can result in improved overall health, enhanced mobility, and an increased quality of life.

Improved Obesity-Related Health Conditions: One of the most remarkable benefits of gastric sleeve surgery is its positive impact on obesity-related health conditions. Many individuals see remarkable improvements in conditions such as type 2 diabetes, high blood pressure, sleep apnea, and high cholesterol. These illnesses may even go into remission in specific circumstances.

Reduced Hunger and Appetite: Gastric sleeve surgery removes a significant portion of the stomach, including the part responsible for producing ghrelin, the hunger hormone. As a result, patients often experience a reduced appetite and fewer cravings for high-calorie foods, making it easier to adhere to a healthier diet.

Minimal Nutritional Concerns: Unlike certain other weight loss surgeries, such as gastric bypass, the gastric sleeve procedure does not involve rerouting the small intestine. Consequently, there is less risk of nutrient malabsorption. While nutritional monitoring and supplementation are essential, the risk of severe deficiencies is lower.

Minimally Invasive Procedure: Gastric sleeve surgery is frequently performed laparoscopically, which means smaller incisions, shorter hospital stays, and quicker recovery times. Minimally invasive surgery generally results in less post-operative pain and fewer complications.

Improved Quality of Life: Achieving significant weight loss and resolving obesity-related health conditions can lead to an improved overall quality of life. Patients often report enhanced energy levels, better physical fitness, and a greater sense of well-being.

Enhanced Body Image and Self-Esteem: The positive impact of weight loss on body image and self-esteem is another valuable benefit. As individuals shed excess weight, they often experience an improved sense of self-confidence and a more positive self-image.

Sustainability: Weight loss achieved through gastric sleeve surgery is often sustainable over the long term. With commitment to a healthy lifestyle, individuals can maintain their progress and continue to enjoy the benefits of weight loss.

Lower Risk of Obesity-Related Complications: Achieving and maintaining a healthier weight can significantly reduce the risk of various obesity-related complications, including heart disease, stroke, certain cancers, and joint problems.

Considerations:

While gastric sleeve surgery offers numerous benefits, it is essential to consider the following aspects:

Permanent Alteration: Gastric sleeve is a permanent procedure. It is not possible to restore the stomach's excised part.
Non-Reversible Decision: Unlike some other weight loss surgeries, such as Lap-Band, the gastric sleeve procedure cannot be reversed.

Nutritional Monitoring: Patients must undergo regular nutritional monitoring and supplementation to ensure they receive essential vitamins and minerals.

Commitment to Lifestyle Changes: To maximize the benefits of gastric sleeve surgery, individuals must be committed to making lasting dietary and lifestyle changes.

Individual Variability: While many individuals experience significant weight loss and health improvements with gastric sleeve, individual results can vary. The degree of weight loss and the resolution of health conditions may differ.

Possible Risks and Complications of Gastric Sleeve Surgery

Gastric sleeve surgery is a highly effective weight loss procedure, but like any surgical intervention, it comes with potential risks and complications. While the benefits often outweigh the drawbacks, individuals considering gastric sleeve surgery should be aware of the potential adverse outcomes and work closely with their healthcare team to minimize these risks. In this chapter, we will explore some of the possible risks and complications associated with gastric sleeve surgery.

Infection: As with any surgical procedure, there is a risk of infection at the incision sites or within the abdominal cavity. Surgical hygiene and proper post-operative wound care can help mitigate this risk.

Bleeding: Some individuals may experience bleeding during or after surgery. This risk is typically managed during the procedure, but postoperative bleeding may require additional intervention or even a return to the operating room.

Leakage: Gastric sleeve surgery involves stapling and suturing the stomach. In rare cases, these staples or sutures can fail, leading to leakage from the stomach into the abdominal cavity. This is a serious complication that may require immediate surgical correction.

Stenosis: Stenosis, or narrowing of the stomach opening, can make it difficult for food to pass from the smaller stomach pouch into the rest of the digestive system. This may cause discomfort, vomiting, and difficulty eating.

Gastroesophageal Reflux Disease (GERD): Some individuals may experience or develop GERD after gastric sleeve surgery. This condition involves the backward flow of stomach acid into the esophagus, leading to heartburn and other symptoms.

Vitamin and Nutrient Deficiencies: Although gastric sleeve surgery has fewer nutritional concerns than some other weight loss procedures, there is still a risk of vitamin and nutrient deficiencies. Patients must commit to lifelong supplementation and regular monitoring of their nutrient levels.

Dumping Syndrome: Dumping syndrome can occur when high-sugar or high-fat foods pass too quickly into the small intestine. It can lead to symptoms such as nausea, diarrhea, and weakness.

Inadequate Weight Loss: While gastric sleeve surgery is highly effective for most individuals, there is a possibility of not achieving the desired weight loss. This can occur if patients do not adhere to the recommended dietary and lifestyle changes.

Reflux or Heartburn: In some cases, gastric sleeve surgery may lead to an increase in reflux symptoms or heartburn. This can be managed with lifestyle modifications or medication.

Gallstones: Rapid weight loss after surgery can increase the risk of gallstones. This may necessitate the removal of the gallbladder in some cases.

Stricture: Stricture is the narrowing of the stomach sleeve, which can cause difficulties in eating and may require treatment, including dilation or reoperation.

Psychological Challenges: Weight loss surgery can bring about emotional and psychological challenges, including body image concerns, depression, or anxiety. It's essential for patients to have access to support services to address these issues.

Long-term Maintenance: Sustaining weight loss and the benefits of surgery requires a lifelong commitment to dietary and lifestyle changes. Failure to do so may lead to weight regain.

Personal Stories and Testimonials

Real-life stories and testimonials from individuals who have undergone gastric sleeve surgery offer powerful insights into the life-changing effects of this procedure. These stories reflect the physical, emotional, and psychological transformations that individuals experience on their journeys to better health. Here are a few compelling narratives that shed light on the diverse experiences of those who have taken the path of gastric sleeve surgery.

Sarah's Gastric Sleeve Journey

Sarah's weight loss journey began with an emotional battle that persisted for years. Struggling with severe obesity, she faced numerous health issues and a significant decline in her quality of life. After exhausting multiple diets and exercise regimens, Sarah decided to explore bariatric surgery as a potential solution. She chose gastric sleeve surgery, and her journey has since transformed her life in remarkable ways.

The Turning Point:

Sarah's turning point came when she realized how her obesity was affecting her health. She was diagnosed with type 2 diabetes and had to rely on multiple medications to manage her condition. Her doctor emphasized the importance of weight loss in controlling her diabetes, and this prompted Sarah to take action.

Choosing Gastric Sleeve Surgery:

After careful research and consultations with healthcare professionals, Sarah opted for gastric sleeve surgery. She was drawn to the procedure's significant weight loss potential and its lower risk of nutritional deficiencies compared to other weight loss surgeries.

The Surgery:

Sarah's surgery went smoothly, and she was back on her feet within a few weeks. The recovery process was challenging at times, but she remained committed to her new path to health.

The Weight Loss Journey:

In the first year following her surgery, Sarah lost over 80 pounds, and her type 2 diabetes went into remission. Her energy levels soared, and she felt more confident than ever. Sarah's wardrobe changed, but more importantly, so did her mindset.

Improved Health and Quality of Life:

Sarah's story is not just about weight loss. It's about reclaiming her life. She no longer relies on diabetes medication, and her blood pressure has normalized. Her joint pain has subsided, and she can now enjoy activities she once avoided.

Support and Determination:

Sarah emphasizes that her support system played a vital role in her success. She joined a support group and connected with people who understood her journey. Sarah's determination to maintain a healthy lifestyle also played a significant part in her success. She now follows a balanced diet, exercises regularly, and embraces a more active lifestyle.

Inspiring Others:

Sarah's journey has inspired many in her community to consider weight loss surgery as a viable solution to obesity and its health-related challenges. She often shares her story in local support groups and online forums, offering guidance and hope to those at the beginning of their own journeys.

Emma's Weight Loss Triumph:

Emma had struggled with obesity since her childhood. She decided to undergo gastric sleeve surgery after numerous attempts to lose weight through diets and exercise. Her journey was not without challenges, but Emma's commitment to her new lifestyle was unwavering. She not only lost a significant amount of weight but also resolved her type 2 diabetes and regained her self-esteem. Emma's story is an inspiration to others who are battling obesity and related health issues.

John's Health Rebirth:

John was in his mid-40s when he opted for gastric sleeve surgery to address his severe obesity. The surgery not only resulted in substantial weight loss but also brought about an incredible transformation in his health. John's high blood pressure and sleep apnea were resolved, and he could finally participate in physical activities he had missed for years. His story is a testament to the life-saving potential of bariatric surgery.

Maria's Emotional Journey:

Maria's gastric sleeve surgery journey was not only about physical changes but also emotional growth. She faced challenges adapting to her new dietary habits and contending with moments of self-doubt. Through it all, Maria developed resilience and learned to prioritize her mental well-being. Her journey highlights the importance of addressing emotional aspects and embracing self-compassion throughout the weight loss process.

David's Support System:

David's story emphasizes the role of a strong support system. He found unwavering support from his partner, friends, and bariatric support groups. Their encouragement, understanding, and shared experiences made a profound difference in his journey to a healthier life. David's narrative is a reminder of the significance of surrounding oneself with people who believe in the pursuit of better health.

Emily's Post-Surgery Lifestyle:

After her gastric sleeve surgery, Emily dedicated herself to adopting a healthier lifestyle. She embraced regular exercise, monitored her nutritional intake, and enjoyed the benefits of her renewed energy. Emily's journey showcases the significance of consistent, long-term commitment to maintaining the results of weight loss surgery.

Michael's Weight Loss and Self-Confidence:

Michael's gastric sleeve surgery journey led to remarkable weight loss and an incredible boost in self-confidence. He shared his story through a blog and social media to inspire others. Michael's experiences show the profound impact that improved self-esteem and a positive self-image can have on one's overall well-being.

Gastric Bypass Surgery

Gastric bypass surgery, known as Roux-en-Y gastric bypass, is a bariatric procedure designed to help individuals achieve significant weight loss while also addressing obesity-related health conditions. This chapter provides a comprehensive overview of gastric bypass surgery, exploring the procedure, benefits, considerations, and potential risks associated with this weight loss surgery.

Procedure:

Gastric bypass surgery is a complex surgical procedure that combines two fundamental mechanisms of weight loss: restriction and malabsorption. The surgery unfolds as follows:

Stomach Pouch Creation: The surgeon begins by stapling off a small, egg-sized pouch at the top of the stomach. This pouch significantly limits the volume of food a person can consume in one sitting.

Small Intestine Rerouting: Following the creation of the stomach pouch, a section of the small intestine is rerouted to connect directly to the pouch. This process bypasses the lower part of the stomach and the upper part of the small intestine, which is primarily responsible for nutrient and calorie absorption.

Benefits of Gastric Bypass Surgery

Gastric bypass surgery, also known as Roux-en-Y gastric bypass, offers a range of profound benefits for individuals struggling with obesity and related health issues. This bariatric procedure has been transformative for many patients, providing them with not only significant weight loss but also improvements in their overall well-being. The numerous benefits of gastric bypass surgery:

Substantial Weight Loss: One of the most notable benefits of gastric bypass surgery is the substantial weight loss it facilitates. Patients often experience an average weight loss of 60% to 80% of their excess body weight within the first year. This weight loss is generally sustained over the long term, significantly improving overall health and mobility.

Resolution of Obesity-Related Health Conditions: Gastric bypass surgery frequently leads to the resolution or significant improvement of obesity-related health issues, including type 2 diabetes, high blood pressure, sleep apnea, and high cholesterol. Many

Patients experience a remarkable turnaround in these conditions, reducing or eliminating the need for medications and enhancing their overall health.

Enhanced Quality of Life: With significant weight loss and improved health comes a noticeable enhancement in the overall quality of life. Patients often report increased energy levels, better physical fitness, and a greater sense of well-being. They can engage in physical activities and social interactions that were previously challenging or impossible.

Reduction in Hunger: Gastric bypass surgery is unique in its ability to reduce hunger significantly. This reduction is attributed to changes in gut hormones that regulate appetite. As a result, patients experience less frequent and intense hunger, making it easier to adhere to healthier eating habits.

Low Risk of Weight Regain: The combination of gastric restriction and malabsorption makes it more challenging for patients to regain substantial amounts of weight after surgery. This lowers the risk of weight regain compared to restrictive procedures alone.

Long-Term Success: Gastric bypass surgery often provides long-lasting weight loss results. With a commitment to a healthy lifestyle, individuals can maintain their progress and continue to enjoy the benefits of weight loss.

Positive Impact on Mental Health: Weight loss through gastric bypass surgery can have a profound impact on mental health. Many patients report an improved self-esteem, body image, and overall mental well-being. This positive change in mental health is often as significant as the physical benefits.

Reduced Risk of Obesity-Related Complications: Achieving and maintaining a healthier weight can significantly reduce the risk of various obesity-related complications, including heart disease, stroke, certain cancers, and joint problems.

Lifestyle Changes: Gastric bypass surgery necessitates long-term commitment to dietary and lifestyle changes. This can lead to improved dietary habits, regular exercise, and a focus on long-term health.

Reduced Medication Dependency: As weight loss and health improvements occur, many patients find that they can reduce or discontinue medications that were previously required to manage obesity-related health conditions.

Considerations:

While gastric bypass surgery offers significant benefits, it is essential to consider the following factors:

Complex Procedure: Gastric bypass is a more complex surgery than some other weight loss procedures, and it requires a high level of surgical expertise.

Nutritional Concerns: The procedure can lead to nutritional deficiencies, particularly in vitamins and minerals. Lifelong monitoring and supplementation are necessary to ensure adequate nutrient intake.

Invasive Nature: Gastric bypass surgery is invasive, involving more substantial incisions and a longer recovery period compared to some other bariatric procedures.

Permanent Alteration: The surgery permanently alters the digestive system, and the changes cannot be reversed.

Commitment to Lifestyle Changes: To achieve and maintain the best results, individuals must commit to making permanent dietary and lifestyle changes.

Individual Variability: Weight loss and health improvements can vary from person to person, and individual outcomes may differ.

Potential Risks and Complications of Gastric Bypass Surgery

While gastric bypass surgery offers significant benefits, like any surgical procedure, it comes with potential risks and complications. Individuals considering this weight loss surgery should be aware of these risks and work closely with their healthcare team to minimize potential adverse outcomes.

Let's explore some of the potential risks and complications associated with gastric bypass surgery.

Infection: There is a risk of infection at the surgical site or within the abdominal cavity. Adhering to strict post-operative hygiene and proper
Wound care can help mitigate this risk.

Bleeding: Some individuals may experience bleeding during or after surgery. While surgical teams are prepared to manage this risk, post-operative bleeding may require additional intervention or even a return to the operating room.

Leakage: Gastric bypass surgery involves reconnecting the small intestine, and in rare cases, this connection can fail, leading to leakage of stomach contents into the abdominal cavity. This is a serious complication that may require immediate surgical correction.

Stricture: Stenosis, or narrowing of the stomach or intestinal opening, can make it difficult for food to pass from the smaller stomach pouch into the rest of the digestive system. This may cause discomfort, vomiting, and difficulty eating.

Gastroesophageal Reflux Disease (GERD): Some individuals may experience or develop GERD after gastric bypass surgery. This condition involves the backward flow of stomach acid into the esophagus, leading to heartburn and other symptoms.

Dumping Syndrome: Dumping syndrome can occur when high-sugar or high-fat foods pass too quickly into the small intestine. This can lead to symptoms such as nausea, diarrhea, and weakness.

Vitamin and Nutrient Deficiencies: Gastric bypass surgery significantly reduces nutrient absorption. Patients must commit to lifelong monitoring and supplementation to prevent nutritional deficiencies. Common deficiencies include vitamins (such as B12, D, and folic acid) and minerals (such as iron and calcium).

Stomal Ulcers: Ulcers can develop at the site where the stomach pouch and small intestine are connected, known as the stoma. These ulcers can cause pain, bleeding, or discomfort.

Gallstones: Following surgery, a rapid weight loss may raise the risk of gallstones. This may necessitate the removal of the gallbladder in some cases.

Stenosis: Stenosis or narrowing of the stomach pouch or intestinal connection can cause difficulties in eating and may require treatment, including dilation or reoperation.

Psychological Challenges: Weight loss surgery can bring about emotional and psychological challenges, including body image concerns, depression, or anxiety. It's essential for patients to have access to support services to address these issues.

Long-Term Maintenance: Sustaining weight loss and the benefits of surgery requires a lifelong commitment to dietary and lifestyle changes. Failure to do so may lead to weight regain.

Personal Stories and Testimonials

Mark's Journey with Gastric Bypass Surgery

Mark's battle with obesity had been a long and arduous one. As his weight continued to impact his health and quality of life, he knew he needed to make a significant change. He decided to undergo gastric bypass surgery to regain control of his health and future.

The Decision to Change

Mark's journey began with the decision to undergo gastric bypass surgery. "It wasn't an easy decision, but I knew it was the right one for me," he says. The support of his family and healthcare team provided the encouragement he needed to take this life-altering step.

Preparation and Surgery

The days leading up to surgery were filled with anticipation and preparation. Mark's healthcare team guided him through the preoperative process, helping him get mentally and physically ready for the procedure.

The surgery itself was a significant event, but Mark's determination to improve his health made it feel like the first step toward a brighter future.

Early Days Post-Surgery

The immediate post-surgery period presented some challenges as Mark's body adjusted to the changes. "The first few weeks were tough, but I kept reminding myself why I had chosen this path," he shares. Adhering to the prescribed diet and gradually reintroducing foods were crucial in ensuring a smooth recovery.

Health Transformation

As the weeks passed, Mark began to see significant changes. "The weight started coming off, and my energy levels increased," he says with a smile. Alongside the physical changes, he also noticed improvements in his health. "a time ago I relied on medications for high blood pressure and diabetes, but as I lost some weight, my doctor was able to adjust my medications," he says.

Embracing a New Lifestyle

Mark's post-surgery journey wasn't just about weight loss; it was about embracing a new lifestyle. He focused on nourishing his body with healthy foods and regular exercise, transforming his relationship with food and physical activity.

Support and Gratitude

Mark emphasizes the importance of support throughout his journey. Having a solid support network was crucial, both from my family and my medical team. They supported me at every turn," he explains.

Today, Mark is thriving. He has achieved and maintained a significant weight loss and is enjoying an improved quality of life. "The procedure for a gastric bypass was the starting point for my change.," he reviews. "It gave me the opportunity to take charge of my health and create a brighter future."

Laura's Weight Loss Journey:

Laura's struggle with obesity had persisted for years. She decided to undergo gastric bypass surgery as a life-changing step towards improved health. Over the course of a year, she achieved remarkable weight loss, losing

75% of her excess body weight. Laura not only regained her self-confidence but also experienced the resolution of her type 2 diabetes and high blood pressure. Her journey is a testament to the life-saving potential of bariatric surgery.

Mark's Transformation:

Mark's decision to undergo gastric bypass surgery was motivated by a desire to overcome his obesity-related health conditions. With the support of his healthcare team, he embarked on this life-changing journey. Within the first year, he lost over 100 pounds, resulting in the resolution of his sleep apnea and a significant improvement in his quality of life. Mark's story is a source of inspiration for individuals seeking a healthier future.

Michelle's Emotional Evolution:

For Michelle, the journey through gastric bypass surgery was as much about emotional growth as it was about physical change. Adapting to new dietary habits and facing moments of self-doubt challenged her, but she learned to prioritize her mental well-being. Her journey underscores the importance of addressing emotional aspects and embracing self-compassion on the path to better health.

Thomas's Path to Support:

Thomas's journey through gastric bypass surgery was significantly enriched by the unwavering support of his spouse, friends, and fellow bariatric support group members. Their encouragement, understanding, and shared experiences made a profound difference in his transition to a healthier life. Thomas's story emphasizes the significance of surrounding oneself with people who believe in the pursuit of better health.

Sarah's Post-Surgery Lifestyle:

After her gastric bypass surgery, Sarah committed herself to adopting a healthier lifestyle. She embraced regular exercise, monitored her nutritional intake, and enjoyed the benefits of her renewed energy. Sarah's journey showcases the importance of consistent, long-term commitment to maintaining the results of weight loss surgery.

Robert's Boost in Self-Confidence:

Robert's gastric bypass journey not only led to substantial weight loss but also provided a remarkable boost in self-esteem. His transformation inspired him to share his experiences through a blog, offering encouragement and motivation to others. Robert's story underscores the profound impact that an improved self-image and increased self-confidence can have on overall well-being.

Choosing the Right Weight Loss Surgery Procedure

Selecting the most suitable weight loss surgery procedure is a crucial decision on your path to a healthier and more fulfilling life. Remember that there is no one-size-fits-all solution. The right weight loss surgery procedure for one person may not be the best choice for another. There are several options available, including gastric bypass, gastric sleeve, and others. Making an informed choice involves considering your individual circumstances, health goals, and the guidance of your healthcare team.

Factors in the Decision-Making Process for Weight Loss Surgery

The decision to undergo weight loss surgery is a significant and often life-changing choice. It involves careful consideration of various factors to ensure the selected procedure aligns with individual needs and goals. Here, we explore the key factors that play a pivotal role in the decision-making process for weight loss surgery.

1. Health and Medical Considerations:

Body Mass Index (BMI): Your BMI is a crucial factor in determining eligibility for weight loss surgery and influences the choice of procedure. Different procedures may be recommended based on your BMI.

Obesity-Related Health Conditions: The presence and severity of obesity-related health conditions, such as type 2 diabetes, high blood pressure, sleep apnea, and joint issues, will impact the decision-making process. Some surgeries are more effective in resolving specific health issues.

Overall Health Status: Your overall health, including any medical conditions unrelated to obesity, is a critical consideration. Pre-existing health conditions can affect the safety and appropriateness of specific procedures.

2. Weight Loss Goals and Expectations:

Weight Loss Expectations: Clarify your weight loss goals. Are you seeking to achieve a specific amount of weight loss, resolve obesity-related health conditions, or improve overall quality of life? Different procedures may offer varying levels of weight loss.

Timeline: Consider your expectations regarding the timeline for weight loss. Some procedures result in more rapid initial weight loss, while others offer slower but steady progress.

3. Lifestyle Commitment:

Commitment to Dietary and Lifestyle Changes: Weight loss surgery requires a lifelong commitment to dietary modifications, regular physical activity, and adherence to post-operative guidelines. Evaluate your readiness to make and sustain these changes.

4. Nutritional Considerations:

Nutritional Deficiencies: Different procedures carry varying risks of nutritional deficiencies. Understanding these risks and committing to lifelong monitoring and supplementation is essential.

5. Surgical Risks and Complications:

Risks and Complications: Discuss the potential risks and complications associated with each procedure with your healthcare team. Consider the impact these risks may have on your decision.

6. Age and Overall Health:

Age: Your age is a factor in the decision-making process. Certain surgeries may be more suitable for younger individuals, while others may be preferred for older patients.

7. Psychological and Emotional Readiness:

Mental Health and Emotional Preparedness: Assess your psychological and emotional readiness for weight loss surgery. Some procedures may have specific emotional considerations.

8. Support System:

Support Network: The support system you have in place can play a significant role in your success. Evaluate the strength of your support system, including family, friends, and bariatric support groups.

9. Personal Preferences:

Personal Comfort and Preference: Consider your personal comfort and confidence with each procedure. It's essential to choose a surgery that aligns with your preferences.

10. Cost and Insurance Coverage:

Financial Considerations: Evaluate the cost of the procedure and whether it is covered by your health insurance. It's critical to comprehend the financial implications of weight loss surgery.

Weight Loss Goals and Expectations in Weight Loss Surgery

Setting clear weight loss goals and managing expectations are fundamental steps in the weight loss surgery journey. It's important to establish realistic and achievable objectives, as this will guide the choice of procedure and help individuals stay motivated throughout their transformation. Here, we will delve into the significance of setting weight loss goals and understanding what to expect when considering weight loss surgery.

1. Defining Your Weight Loss Goals:

When considering weight loss surgery, it's essential to define your specific weight loss goals. These objectives will serve as a roadmap and provide clarity throughout your journey. Consider the following factors:

Desired Weight: What is your target weight or desired weight range? Discuss this with your healthcare team to ensure that your goals are realistic and achievable.

Percentage of Excess Weight: Many weight loss goals are expressed as a percentage of excess body weight. For instance, some individuals aim to lose 50% or 75% of their excess weight.

Health-Related Goals: Are there specific health goals you wish to achieve, such as resolving type 2 diabetes, improving mobility, or managing high blood pressure?

Improving Quality of Life: Consider how weight loss will enhance your overall quality of life. This may include being more active, enjoying a better social life, or boosting your self-esteem.

2. Realistic Expectations:

Managing expectations is vital in the weight loss surgery process. Recognize that while surgery can be transformative, it is not a magic solution. Consider the following to set realistic expectations:

Gradual Weight Loss: Weight loss after surgery typically occurs gradually. It may take months to reach your target weight, and the pace can vary among individuals.

Non-Linear Progress: Weight loss is not always linear. Plateaus and periods of slower progress can be part of the journey.

Lifestyle Changes: Understand that surgery is just one part of the equation. Committing to dietary modifications, regular physical activity, and adherence to post-operative guidelines are essential for success.

Possible Plateaus and Challenges: Expect that you may encounter plateaus or face challenges in maintaining a healthy lifestyle. These are normal aspects of the journey.

3. Health Improvements:

While weight loss is a significant goal, remember that health improvements are equally vital. Many individuals choose weight loss surgery to resolve obesity-related health conditions. Ensure your expectations include the potential for improved health, such as the remission of type 2 diabetes or better management of high blood pressure.

4. Monitoring Progress:

Regularly monitoring your progress and staying engaged with your healthcare team is crucial. They can help you set realistic expectations and provide guidance based on your individual health profile.

5. Support and Accountability:

A strong support system can play a pivotal role in managing expectations and achieving your goals. Engaging with support groups, friends, and family members who understand your journey can provide motivation and accountability.

Medical History and Pre-existing Conditions in Weight Loss Surgery

Your medical history and pre-existing conditions play a pivotal role in the decision to undergo weight loss surgery. Understanding your health background is crucial for assessing your eligibility for surgery, determining the most appropriate procedure, and ensuring a safe and successful outcome. In this chapter, we explore the significance of medical history and pre-existing conditions when considering weight loss surgery.

1. Medical History Assessment:

When you contemplate weight loss surgery, your healthcare team will conduct a comprehensive evaluation of your medical history. This assessment typically includes:

Pre-existing Conditions: Any chronic health conditions you currently have, such as type 2 diabetes, high blood pressure, sleep apnea, or joint problems, will be evaluated.

Previous Surgeries and Medical Interventions: Details of any prior surgeries, medical procedures, or interventions are important, as they can influence the choice of weight loss procedure.

Medications and Allergies: Your current medications and any allergies you have will be assessed to ensure that your surgical plan is safe and compatible with your existing health regimen.

Family Medical History: A family medical history is also relevant, as it can provide insight into potential genetic factors that might influence your health.

2. Impact on Weight Loss Surgery Eligibility:

Your medical history can influence your eligibility for weight loss surgery. Conditions such as uncontrolled psychiatric illnesses, active substance abuse, certain autoimmune diseases, and specific heart conditions may affect your suitability for surgery. Your healthcare team will help you determine whether you meet the criteria for weight loss surgery based on your medical history.

3. Procedure Selection:

Certain pre-existing conditions may influence the choice of weight loss procedure. For example, individuals with severe acid reflux might be directed toward procedures that reduce acid reflux, such as a gastric bypass. Conversely, those without such issues might opt for a gastric sleeve procedure. Your medical history will guide your healthcare team in recommending the most appropriate surgery.

4.   Post-Operative   Health Management:

If you have pre-existing conditions, your healthcare team will work with you to develop a post-operative plan for managing and monitoring these conditions. This may involve adjustments to medications, changes in lifestyle, or additional post-operative support.

5. Health Improvements:

The resolution or improvement of pre-existing conditions is a common motivation for undergoing weight loss surgery. Many patients experience positive changes in their health after surgery, such as the remission of type 2 diabetes, better blood pressure control, and improved sleep apnea. These potential health improvements are a significant incentive for individuals with pre-existing conditions.

6. Ongoing Health Monitoring:

Continual monitoring of your health is essential. Regular check-ups, follow-up appointments with your healthcare team, and adherence to prescribed post-operative guidelines are vital for maintaining and optimizing the improvements in your health achieved through weight loss surgery.

7. Personalized Guidance:

Every individual's medical history and pre-existing conditions are unique. Therefore, the guidance and support provided by your healthcare team should be personalized to your specific health profile. They will work with you to create a plan that addresses your individual needs and goals.

Lifestyle Considerations in Weight Loss Surgery

Weight loss surgery is not just a medical procedure; it's a transformative journey that involves significant lifestyle changes. These changes are essential for achieving and maintaining a healthier weight and improving overall well-being. In this chapter, we explore the lifestyle considerations that are crucial before and after weight loss surgery.

1. Pre-Operative Lifestyle Considerations:

Before undergoing weight loss surgery, individuals should prepare by making the following lifestyle adjustments:

Dietary Habits: Begin transitioning to a healthier diet by reducing high-calorie, high-sugar, and high-fat foods. This helps prepare your body for the changes it will undergo post-surgery.

Portion Control: Practice portion control and mindful eating. Learning to eat smaller meals and stop when satisfied is an important skill for post-surgery success.

Hydration: Stay well-hydrated by drinking plenty of water. Proper hydration is essential for overall health and is equally important after surgery.

Physical Activity: Start incorporating regular physical activity into your routine. Building a foundation of fitness can improve your recovery and make it easier to embrace an active lifestyle post-surgery.

Behavioral Changes: Address emotional eating and unhealthy food-related behaviors. Seek support from a therapist or counselor if needed to prepare for the emotional aspects of weight loss.

2.   Post-Operative   Lifestyle Considerations:

After weight loss surgery, there are several lifestyle considerations that are crucial for success:

Dietary Modifications: You'll need to follow a specific post-operative diet that gradually progresses from liquids to solid foods. Adhering to these guidelines is essential for a successful recovery and long-term weight loss.

Portion Control: Continue to practice portion control, as your stomach's capacity will be significantly reduced after surgery.

Nutritional Supplements: Ensure you take prescribed nutritional supplements to prevent deficiencies in vitamins and minerals, as absorption may be compromised.

Regular Exercise: Commit to regular exercise. Engaging in physical activity not only enhances weight loss but also improves overall health and well-being.

Hydration: Maintain proper hydration post-surgery. Adequate water intake is crucial for overall health and aids in weight loss.

Lifestyle Accountability: Seek the support of a bariatric support group or therapist to help you address emotional and behavioral aspects of your relationship with food. Lifestyle accountability is vital for long-term success.

Social and Family Support: Engage your family and friends in your journey to healthier living. Their support can be invaluable.

Frequent Follow-Up Appointments: Show up for all of your planned follow-up visits with your medical team. These appointments are important for monitoring your progress and addressing any concerns.

3. Emotional and Psychological Considerations:

Lifestyle changes often come with emotional and psychological challenges. It's crucial to:

- Deal with emotional eating and create constructive coping mechanisms.
- Embrace a positive self-image and self-compassion as you experience physical changes.

- Seek support from mental health professionals or bariatric support groups to navigate the emotional aspects of weight loss.

4. Long-Term Commitment:

Weight loss surgery is a lifelong commitment. It's essential to understand that maintaining a healthier weight and enjoying the benefits of the surgery require ongoing dedication to the lifestyle changes mentioned above.

5. Personalized Guidance:

Lifestyle considerations are highly individual, and your healthcare team will provide personalized guidance to ensure your journey is tailored to your specific needs and goals.

Preparing for Weight Loss Surgery

Preparing for weight loss surgery is a multifaceted process that involves physical, mental, and logistical considerations. Effective preparation for weight loss surgery involves a combination of medical assessments, lifestyle changes, mental readiness, and logistical planning. Engaging with your healthcare team and building a support network are essential components of a successful journey.

Medical Evaluations and Consultations for Weight Loss Surgery

Medical evaluations and consultations are integral components of the weight loss surgery journey. These assessments help determine your eligibility for surgery, select the most appropriate procedure, and ensure a safe and successful outcome. Here, we will delve into the significance of medical evaluations and consultations in the context of weight loss surgery.

1. Initial Consultation:

Meet with a Bariatric Surgeon: The journey begins with an initial consultation with a qualified bariatric surgeon. During this meeting, you'll discuss your medical history, health goals, and reasons for considering weight loss surgery. It's an opportunity to ask questions and gain an understanding of the process.

2. Comprehensive Medical Evaluation:

Review of Medical History: Your medical history will be looked into in detail. This includes past and current medical conditions, surgeries, medications, allergies, and family medical history.

Physical Examination: A physical examination may be conducted to assess your current health and any obesity-related conditions.

Diagnostic Tests: Your healthcare team may recommend diagnostic tests, such as blood work, imaging (e.g., X-rays or ultrasounds), and cardiac evaluations to assess your overall health.

3. Psychological Assessment:

Psychological Evaluation: A psychological assessment is often part of the pre-operative process. It helps identify any emotional or behavioral factors that could impact your success post-surgery. This evaluation may include interviews, questionnaires, and discussions with a mental health professional.

4. Procedure Selection:

Procedure Discussion: Based on your medical evaluation and your health goals, your surgeon will discuss the most appropriate weight loss procedure for your individual circumstances. Factors such as your BMI, medical history, and health conditions will influence this decision.

5. Informed Consent:

Understanding Risks and Benefits: Your surgeon will provide you with detailed information about the risks and benefits of weight loss surgery. You will be required to provide informed consent, indicating that you understand the procedure and its potential outcomes.

6. Pre-operative Diet and Lifestyle Guidance:

Dietary and Lifestyle Counseling: You'll receive guidance on pre-operative dietary and lifestyle changes. This may include adjusting your eating habits, reducing calorie intake, practicing portion control, and increasing physical activity.

7. Personalized Plan:

Individualized Care: Your healthcare team will create an individualized care plan based on the information gathered during the medical evaluations and consultations. This plan outlines the steps you need to take in preparation for surgery and the necessary support you'll receive during your journey.

8. Financial and Insurance Guidance:

Financial Considerations: Consult with your healthcare team or hospital administrators to understand the financial aspects of weight loss surgery. This includes assessing your insurance coverage and identifying any out-of-pocket costs.

9. Support System:

Building a Support Network: Engage your family and friends in your journey. Their support is invaluable. Additionally, consider joining a bariatric support group or an online community to connect with others who have undergone similar experiences.

Dietary Changes and Pre-Operative Diet for Weight Loss Surgery

Dietary changes are a fundamental aspect of preparing for weight loss surgery. These changes serve several purposes, including reducing liver size, helping with post-operative recovery, and setting the stage for long-term success. The dietary modifications and the pre-operative diet that are essential in the lead-up to weight loss surgery:

1. Dietary Changes Before Surgery:

Caloric Restriction: Begin reducing your daily caloric intake to create a calorie deficit, which can facilitate weight loss before surgery. This step helps shrink the liver and reduce surgical risks.

Portion Control: Practice portion control and mindful eating. Learning to eat smaller meals and stopping when satisfied is crucial for post-surgery success.

Balanced Nutrition: Prioritize nutrient-dense foods to ensure you are receiving essential vitamins and minerals. Prioritize eating a diet high in fruits, vegetables, whole grains, and lean proteins.

Sugar and Fat Reduction: Gradually reduce the consumption of sugary and high-fat foods. This change can assist in weight loss and promote healthier eating habits.

Hydration: Stay well-hydrated by drinking plenty of water. Proper hydration is crucial for overall health and is equally important before surgery.

Alcohol Reduction: If you consume alcohol, consider reducing your intake. Alcohol can contribute to liver enlargement and should be minimized before surgery.

2. Pre-Operative Diet:

Prescribed Diet Plan: Your healthcare team will provide a specific preoperative diet plan. This plan typically consists of phases, which may include:

Liquid Diet: A phase during which you will consume clear liquids and protein shakes. This phase is intended to further reduce liver size and prepare the digestive system.

Full Liquid Diet: This phase introduces thicker liquids and soft foods, such as soups and purees.

Solid Foods: A gradual reintroduction of solid foods while continuing to focus on high-protein, low-calorie options.

Nutritional Supplements: Your healthcare team may recommend nutritional supplements to ensure you receive essential vitamins and minerals. Weight loss surgery can impact nutrient absorption, making supplementation crucial.

Elimination of Specific Foods: In the weeks leading up to surgery, your healthcare team may recommend eliminating specific foods that can increase the risk of complications. This often includes foods that are difficult to digest or can lead to digestive discomfort.

3. Personalized Guidance:

Individualized Plans: The dietary changes and pre-operative diet plan will be personalized to your specific health profile and the type of weight loss surgery you will undergo. Your healthcare team will ensure the plan aligns with your unique needs.

4. Nutritional Counseling:

Dietary Guidance: Seek the guidance of a registered dietitian or nutritionist who specializes in bariatric care. They can provide dietary counseling, meal planning, and support throughout your pre-operative journey.

5. Psychological and Emotional Support:

Handle Emotional Eating: It's critical to address emotional eating patterns if you suffer from them before surgery. Consider seeking support from a therapist or counselor who specializes in bariatric mental health.

Emotional Preparedness: Mentally prepare yourself for the changes ahead. Weight loss surgery involves significant dietary and lifestyle adjustments, and it's essential to be emotionally ready for this transformation.

Lifestyle Adjustments for Post-Weight Loss Surgery Success

Weight loss surgery is not merely a medical procedure; it's a transformative journey that necessitates significant lifestyle adjustments. These changes are fundamental for achieving and sustaining a healthier weight and overall well-being. Here, we will explore the key lifestyle adjustments required for a successful post-weight loss surgery experience.

1. Dietary Modifications:

Portion Control: After weight loss surgery, your stomach's capacity will be significantly reduced. Learning portion control is essential to avoid overeating and support your weight loss journey.

High-Protein Diet: Emphasize a high-protein diet to ensure you get adequate nutrition and support muscle maintenance during weight loss.

Nutrient-Dense Foods: Prioritize nutrient-dense foods such as fruits, vegetables, whole grains, and lean proteins. These foods provide essential vitamins and minerals for your health.

Hydration: Stay well-hydrated by drinking water and avoiding sugary beverages. Proper hydration is essential for overall health.

Limit Sugar and Processed Foods: Reduce the consumption of sugary and highly processed foods, which can lead to weight regain and affect your health.

Balanced Meals: Strive for balanced meals that include a variety of food groups to meet your nutritional needs.

2. Regular Physical Activity:

Incorporate Exercise: Regular physical activity is crucial for weight loss, muscle maintenance, and overall well-being. Engage in a workout routine that you enjoy and can sustain.

Consult with a Fitness Professional: Consider working with a fitness professional to develop a personalized exercise plan based on your fitness level and goals.

Progressive Approach: Begin gradually and build up the intensity and duration of your workouts over time.

3. Behavior and Emotional Health:

Counseling Support: Seek assistance from a therapist or counselor who specializes in bariatric mental health if you struggle with emotional eating or harmful food-related habits.

Address Emotional Triggers: Learn to recognize and address emotional triggers for overeating. Create effective coping mechanisms to control stress, worry, and other feelings.

4. Social and Family Support:

Engage Your Support System: Involve your family and friends in your journey to healthier living. Establish useful coping strategies to manage stress, anxiety, and other emotions.

Join Support Groups: Consider joining a bariatric support group or an online community to connect with individuals who have gone through similar experiences.

5. Regular Follow-Up Appointments:

Scheduled Check-Ups: Attend all scheduled follow-up appointments with your healthcare team. These appointments are crucial for monitoring your progress, addressing any concerns, and making necessary adjustments to your plan.

6. Emotional and Psychological Well-Being:

Positive Self-Image: Embrace a positive self-image and practice self-compassion as you experience physical changes. Weight loss surgery can bring about emotional and psychological adjustments, and it's important to develop a healthy self-concept.

Address Emotional Challenges: If you encounter emotional challenges or concerns, reach out to your support network or a mental health professional for assistance.

7. Ongoing Commitment:

Lifelong Dedication: Understand that weight loss surgery is a lifelong commitment. The lifestyle adjustments you make are not temporary but are integral to maintaining a healthier weight and overall well-being.

Addressing Common Concerns in the Weight Loss Surgery Journey

Weight loss surgery is a transformative and life-changing journey that can be accompanied by various concerns and uncertainties. It's important to address these common concerns and questions to ensure a successful and confident journey. Here, we'll explore some of the typical concerns and provide guidance on how to address them.

1. Concerns About Surgical Risks:

Weight loss surgery, like any medical procedure, carries certain risks. To address this concern:

Consult with Your Surgeon: Have open and candid discussions with your bariatric surgeon to understand the specific risks associated with your chosen procedure. Your surgeon can provide detailed information and steps taken to minimize these risks.

Informed Consent: Ensure you have a clear understanding of the procedure and its potential risks. Providing informed consent is a necessary step before surgery.

2. Fear of Pain and Discomfort:

Post-operative pain and discomfort can be a concern. To address this:

Pain Management Plan: Your healthcare team will have a pain management plan in place. They will provide you with appropriate pain relief medication and guidance on post-operative comfort.

Focus on Recovery: Remember that the initial discomfort is temporary, and it is a part of the healing process. The soreness will lessen as you heal.

3. Emotional Concerns:

Weight loss surgery can bring about emotional challenges. To address emotional concerns:

Mental Health Support: Consider seeking support from a therapist or counselor who specializes in bariatric mental health. They can help you navigate the emotional aspects of the journey.

Support Groups: Join a bariatric support group or an online community to connect with others who are going through similar experiences. Sharing your concerns and listening to others can provide emotional support.

4. Fear of Weight Regain:

The fear of regaining weight after surgery is a common concern. To address this:

Commit to Lifestyle Changes: Understand that weight loss surgery is a tool that requires lifelong commitment to dietary and lifestyle changes. Adhering to these changes is key to maintaining your weight loss.

Frequent Follow-Up: Show up for all of your planned follow-up sessions with your medical team. These appointments are essential for monitoring your progress and making necessary adjustments to your plan if needed.

5. Concerns About Nutritional Deficiencies:

Weight loss surgery can impact nutrient absorption, potentially leading to deficiencies. To address this:

Nutritional Supplements: Follow your healthcare team's recommendations for nutritional supplementation to prevent deficiencies.

Regular Monitoring: Your healthcare team will regularly monitor your nutritional status and make adjustments to your supplementation as needed.

6. Social and Family Concerns:

Engaging family and friends in your journey can sometimes be challenging. To address this:

Educate Your Support System: Share information about your surgery and the lifestyle changes you're making with your support system. Educate them about the importance of their support and understanding.

Join Support Groups: Encourage your loved ones to attend support group meetings or connect with other families of bariatric patients to gain insights into the journey.

7. Lifestyle Adjustments:

Adjusting to the lifestyle changes required after surgery can be a concern. To address this:

Gradual Transition: Understand that lifestyle adjustments are gradual. It's a journey, and you'll have time to adapt to your new habits.

Seek Professional Guidance: Consult with a registered dietitian or nutritionist who specializes in bariatric care for personalized dietary advice.

The Surgical Experience in Weight Loss Surgery

The surgical experience in weight loss surgery is a significant step in your transformative journey toward a healthier, happier life. This chapter provides an overview of what you can expect during the surgical process and the postoperative period.

1. Pre-Operative Preparations:

Before the day of your surgery, you will undergo several pre-operative preparations, including:

Final Consultation: You may have a final consultation with your surgeon to address any last-minute questions and concerns.

Fasting: You will be required to fast for a specific period before surgery. Your healthcare team will provide clear instructions.

Hospital Check-In: On the day of surgery, you will check into the hospital or surgical center. You'll be guided through the registration process and taken to the pre-operative area.

Pre-Operative Assessments: You may undergo pre-operative assessments, including a final review of your medical history, vital signs, and preparations for anesthesia.

2. The Surgery Itself:

The specifics of the surgery will depend on the type of weight loss procedure you've chosen (e.g., gastric sleeve, gastric bypass). However, some common elements include:

Anesthesia: You'll be administered general anesthesia, which ensures you are unconscious and pain-free during the surgery.

Surgical Procedure: The surgery will be performed through small incisions (laparoscopic) or, in some cases, an open procedure. Your surgeon will carry out the chosen weight loss procedure, which can take several hours.

Hospital Stay: The duration of your hospital stay may vary, but it generally ranges from one to three days, depending on the type of surgery and your recovery progress.

3. Immediate Post-Operative Recovery:

Recovery Room: After surgery, you will be taken to the recovery room, where you will wake up from anesthesia. You will be closely monitored during this initial postoperative period.

Pain Management: Pain management will be a priority. You may receive pain relief medication as needed.

Fluid Intake: Initially, you will not be allowed to drink or eat, as your digestive system needs time to heal.

4. Transition to a New Diet:

Liquid Diet: Your healthcare team will gradually introduce liquids and then soft foods in the days following surgery. This diet progression is closely monitored to ensure proper healing.

5. Post-Operative Care:

Pain Management: Pain management continues as you recover. Your healthcare team will provide guidance on managing discomfort.

Monitoring: You will be monitored for any signs of complications, and your healthcare team will perform regular checks on your vital signs and overall health.

6. Hospital Discharge:

Once your healthcare team determines that you are ready for discharge, you will receive instructions for your recovery at home. This typically includes guidance on diet, activity, medications, and follow-up appointments.

7. Recovery at Home:

The initial recovery at home involves:

Diet Adherence: Strict adherence to the prescribed diet is essential for a successful recovery.

Activity Gradual Increase: Gradually increase your physical activity according to your surgeon's recommendations.

Medications: Take any prescribed medications as directed.

Monitoring: Continue to monitor your health and watch for any signs of complications.

8. Follow-Up Appointments:

You will have a series of follow-up appointments with your healthcare team to monitor your progress and address any questions or concerns. These appointments are crucial for optimizing your recovery and long-term success.

What to Expect on the Day of Weight Loss Surgery

The day of your weight loss surgery is a significant milestone in your journey toward better health and well-being. Understanding what to expect on this day can help alleviate anxiety and ensure a smoother experience. Here, we provide an overview of what you can anticipate on the day of your surgery.

Arrival at the Hospital or Surgical Center:

On the morning of your surgery, you will check into the hospital or surgical center. It's essential to arrive on time, so plan your transportation accordingly.

Registration and Paperwork:

Upon arrival, you will complete any necessary paperwork and registration procedures. This may include verifying your identity, confirming insurance information, and signing consent forms.

Change into a Hospital Gown:

There will be a hospital gown available for you to change into. This gown ensures that you wear comfortable, sterile clothing during surgery.

Pre-Operative Assessment:

Your healthcare team will conduct a pre-operative assessment, which typically includes:

- Review of your medical history and medications.
- Measurement of vital signs such as blood pressure, heart rate, and temperature.
- Placement of an intravenous (IV) line to provide fluids and medications.

Pre-Operative Conversations:

You will have conversations with your surgical team, including the surgeon, anesthesiologist, and nurses. This is an opportunity to ask any last-minute questions or express concerns.

Anesthesia Administration:

Before surgery, you will receive general anesthesia, which will put you to sleep and keep you pain-free during the procedure.

The Surgical Procedure:

The specifics of the surgical procedure will depend on the type of weight loss surgery you've chosen (e.g., gastric sleeve, gastric bypass). The surgery can take several hours, during which your surgeon will carry out the necessary steps to complete the procedure.

Recovery in the Post-Anesthesia Care Unit (PACU):

After the surgery, you will be taken to the recovery room, known as the Post-Anesthesia Care Unit (PACU). Here's What to anticipate on the day of surgery for weight loss:

You will wake up from anesthesia. It's normal to feel groggy and disoriented at this stage.

You will be closely monitored by healthcare professionals to ensure you are recovering well and that your vital signs are stable.

You may receive pain relief medication if needed.

Transition to a Hospital Room:

Once your healthcare team determines that you are stable and awake, you will be transferred to a hospital room. The duration of your stay will depend on the type of surgery and your recovery progress.

Post-Operative Recovery:

In your hospital room, you will continue to recover from surgery. Your healthcare team will closely monitor your condition and provide pain management and any necessary medical care.

Introduction to Diet Progression:

Your diet progression will begin in the days following surgery. You will start with clear liquids and then transition to thicker liquids and soft foods. This dietary progression is closely monitored to ensure proper healing.

Preparing for Discharge:

Once your healthcare team determines that you are ready for discharge, you will receive detailed instructions for your recovery at home. This will include guidance on diet, activity, medications, and follow-up appointments.

Anesthesia and Surgery Duration in Weight Loss Surgery

Anesthesia and the duration of the surgical procedure are critical aspects of the weight loss surgery process. Insights of what you can expect regarding anesthesia and the length of the surgery during your weight loss journey.

1. Anesthesia in Weight Loss Surgery:

General Anesthesia: In weight loss surgery, general anesthesia is commonly used. General anesthesia renders you completely unconscious and pain-free during the procedure. It is administered through an intravenous (IV) line and inhaled gasses. While under general anesthesia, you will not be aware of the surgery, and you will not experience pain or discomfort.

Anesthesiologist's Role: An anesthesiologist is a medical doctor who specializes in administering anesthesia and monitoring your vital signs throughout the surgery. They ensure that you are safely asleep and comfortable during the procedure.

Pre-Anesthesia Assessment: Before administering anesthesia, the anesthesiologist will conduct a pre-operative assessment. This assessment includes reviewing your medical history, medications, allergies, and any specific concerns related to anesthesia. It's crucial to provide accurate information during this assessment to ensure your safety.

2. Duration of Weight Loss Surgery:

The duration of weight loss surgery varies depending on the type of procedure you've chosen (e.g., gastric sleeve, gastric bypass) and the specific circumstances of your surgery. Here are some estimates for common weight loss procedures:

Gastric Sleeve (Sleeve Gastrectomy): Gastric sleeve surgery typically takes around 60 to 90 minutes to complete. It involves removing a large portion of the stomach and reshaping the remaining part into a smaller sleeve-like structure.

Gastric Bypass (Roux-en-Y): Gastric bypass surgery generally takes approximately 90 to 120 minutes. This procedure involves creating a smaller stomach pouch and rerouting the small intestine to connect to the pouch. It effectively reduces the amount of food you can eat and alters the digestion process.

Adjustable Gastric Banding (Lap-Band): Adjustable gastric banding surgeries usually take about 30 to 60 minutes. It entails encircling the upper portion of the stomach with an adjustable band to form a smaller pouch.

Biliopancreatic Diversion with Duodenal Switch (BPD/DS): BPD/DS is a complex procedure and can take approximately 120 to 180 minutes or longer. It involves a significant restructuring of the digestive system, including creating a smaller stomach pouch and rerouting the small intestine.

It's important to note that the surgery duration can vary based on factors such as the surgeon's experience, your unique anatomy, and any unforeseen complications that may arise during the procedure.

3. Post-Anesthesia Recovery:

After surgery, you will be transferred to the recovery room, also known as the Post-Anesthesia Care Unit (PACU).

Here, you will gradually wake up from anesthesia under the close supervision of the anesthesia team. You may feel groggy and disoriented initially, but as the effects of anesthesia wear off, you will become more alert. Pain management and monitoring of your vital signs are ongoing during this phase.

The duration of your stay in the PACU can vary, depending on your recovery progress and how quickly you wake up from anesthesia. Once you are stable and awake, you will be transferred to a hospital room or recovery area, where you will continue to recover.

The Role of the Healthcare Team in Weight Loss Surgery

Weight loss surgery is a comprehensive journey that requires the expertise and support of a multidisciplinary healthcare team. This chapter outlines the crucial roles of various healthcare professionals who collaborate to ensure your safety, success, and overall well-being during and after your weight loss surgery.

1. Bariatric Surgeon:

The bariatric surgeon is the key figure in your weight loss surgery journey. Their roles include:

- Evaluating your eligibility for surgery based on your health profile and goals.
- Performing the surgical procedure with precision and expertise.
- Discussing the surgery's risks and benefits and obtaining informed consent.

- Providing post-operative care and monitoring your progress during follow-up appointments.

2. Anesthesiologist:

Anesthesiologists are responsible for administering anesthesia and monitoring your vital signs throughout the surgery. Their roles include:

- Conducting pre-operative assessments to determine the most suitable anesthesia.
- Safely administering anesthesia to ensure you are unconscious and pain-free during surgery.
- Continuously monitoring your condition during surgery to ensure your safety and comfort.

3. Registered Dietitian or Nutritionist:

Registered dietitians or nutritionists specializing in bariatric care play a vital role in your weight loss surgery journey. Their roles include:

- Providing dietary counseling and personalized nutrition plans.
- Guiding you through pre-operative and post-operative diets.
- Addressing nutritional needs and potential deficiencies associated with weight loss surgery.

4. Psychologist or Mental Health Professional:

Mental health professionals who specialize in bariatric care are essential for addressing emotional and psychological aspects of the journey. Their roles include:

- Conducting psychological assessments to identify emotional and behavioral factors.
- Offering support and counseling to help you manage stress, anxiety, and emotional challenges.

- Addressing emotional eating and promoting healthy coping strategies.

5. Nurses and Surgical Team:

Nurses and other surgical team members play crucial roles in the surgical process and post-operative care. Their roles include:

- Assisting the surgeon during the procedure.
- Monitoring your condition in the operating room and recovery room.
- Providing immediate post-operative care, including pain management and vital sign monitoring.
- Offering guidance and education on post-operative care and dietary progression.

6. Physical Therapist and Exercise Specialist:

Physical therapists and exercise specialists help you develop and maintain an appropriate exercise routine. Their roles include:

- Designing personalized exercise plans tailored to your fitness level and goals.
- Assisting with rehabilitation and recovery exercises.
- Encouraging regular physical activity to support weight loss and overall well-being.

7. Support Groups and Social Workers:

- Support groups and social workers offer emotional and social support. Their roles include:
- Connecting you with peer support groups and online communities.

- Addressing social and emotional concerns that may arise during your journey.
- Providing guidance on building a support network with family and friends.

8. Hospital Administrators and Insurance Specialists:

Hospital administrators and insurance specialists assist with the logistical and financial aspects of your surgery. Their roles include:

- Managing hospital registration and administrative processes.
- Assisting in understanding your insurance coverage for weight loss surgery.
- Addressing financial and billing inquiries.

9. Primary Care Physician (PCP):

Your primary care physician is an essential part of your healthcare team. Their roles include:

- Coordinating with the bariatric team and providing necessary medical information.
- Monitoring your general health and addressing any non-bariatric-related medical concerns.

10. Long-Term Follow-Up Team:

The long-term follow-up team, including your bariatric surgeon and dietitian, continues to monitor your progress and provide guidance on maintaining a healthy lifestyle.

Recovery and Post-Op Life in Weight Loss Surgery

Recovery and post-operative life in weight loss surgery mark the beginning of a transformative journey toward a healthier, happier you. This chapter provides an overview of what to expect during the recovery phase and how to navigate your new life following surgery.

The Recovery Period

The recovery period following weight loss surgery is a critical phase in your journey toward improved health and well-being. It's a time when your body heals and adjusts to the changes brought about by the surgery. This chapter provides an overview of what to expect during the recovery period and how to navigate it successfully.

1. Initial Post-Operative Recovery:

The immediate post-operative recovery phase typically takes place in the hospital or surgical center. During this time:

Pain Management: Pain management is a priority to ensure your comfort. You may receive pain relief medication as needed.

Monitoring: Healthcare professionals closely monitor your vital signs, incision sites, and overall health. Regular checks are performed to ensure that you are healing properly and not experiencing any complications.

Clear Liquid Diet: Your diet progression typically begins with clear liquids. You will gradually transition to thicker liquids and soft foods as determined by your surgeon and dietitian. It's essential to follow dietary guidelines carefully during this phase.

Hospital Stay: The duration of your hospital stay will depend on the type of surgery and your recovery progress. Usually, it lasts between one and three days.

2. Transition to Home Recovery:

Once your healthcare team determines that you are ready for discharge, you'll receive instructions for your recovery at home. This is a pivotal step in your journey, and it's important to adhere to post-operative guidelines:

Diet Progression: Continue to follow the dietary progression plan provided by your healthcare team. Gradually reintroduce solid foods as guided by your dietitian. Nutritional supplementation, if recommended, should also be part of your daily routine.

Medications: Take any prescribed medications as directed. These may include pain relief medications, antibiotics, and supplements to prevent nutritional deficiencies.

Activity: Gradually increase your physical activity as directed by your surgeon or physical therapist. Gentle, low-impact activities, such as walking, are often recommended initially. It's essential to follow these recommendations to avoid complications and support a healthy recovery.

Monitoring: Continue to monitor your health and watch for any signs of complications. Look out for symptoms such as persistent pain, fever, nausea, vomiting, or any unusual changes. If you have any concerns or questions, don't hesitate to contact your healthcare team.

3. Follow-Up Appointments:

Regular follow-up appointments with your healthcare team are vital for tracking your progress and addressing any concerns. These appointments generally occur at various intervals over the first year and beyond. During these visits:

- Your surgeon will assess your overall health and weight loss progress. They may also evaluate the condition of your surgical incisions.

- A dietitian will provide guidance on dietary adjustments, ensuring you receive adequate nutrition.

- The surgical team will address any concerns related to your procedure or recovery, providing insights and recommendations.

4. Embracing Lifestyle Changes:

Your recovery period is an excellent time to embrace the lifestyle changes essential for your post-operative life:

Dietary Modifications: Follow the dietary guidelines provided by your dietitian. Pay attention to portion control, focus on high-protein foods, incorporate nutrient-dense options, and maintain proper hydration.

Regular Physical Activity: Introduce regular physical activity into your routine. Exercise gently at first, then progressively up the length and intensity. It's essential to engage in physical activities that you enjoy and can maintain over the long term.

Behavioral and Emotional Health: Address any emotional or behavioral factors that may impact your journey. To manage stress or emotional eating, build appropriate coping mechanisms, and get guidance from a therapist or counselor if necessary.

Positive Self-Image: As your body undergoes significant changes, it's important to embrace a positive self-image and practice self-compassion. Developing a healthy self-concept is essential during this transformative period.

5. Ongoing Commitment:

Weight loss surgery is a lifelong commitment. To maintain a healthier weight and overall well-being, you must adhere to dietary and lifestyle changes and maintain consistent follow-up care with your healthcare team.

6. Support System:

Engage your support network, including family and friends. Their understanding and encouragement are invaluable. To make connections with people who have gone through similar things, think about joining support groups or online forums.

Post-Operative Diets and Nutrition in Weight Loss Surgery

Post-operative diets and nutrition play a central role in the success of weight loss surgery. Here, we provide insights into the dietary guidelines, nutritional considerations, and dietary progression you can expect during the post-operative phase of your journey.

Clear Liquid Diet:

Immediately following weight loss surgery, you will begin with a clear liquid diet. This diet progression is typically followed:

Days 1-2: Clear liquids such as water, broth, and sugar-free gelatin. The goal is to stay hydrated and provide essential fluids while allowing your digestive system to rest.

Full Liquid Diet:

After the clear liquid phase, you will transition to a full liquid diet, which includes:

Days 3-14: Protein-rich liquid supplements, thin soups, milk, yogurt, and protein shakes. These options provide essential nutrients, including protein, while maintaining a smooth texture for easy digestion.

Pureed Diet:

The next phase is the pureed diet, which includes:

Weeks 2-4: Pureed or blended foods such as soft fruits, cooked vegetables, and lean protein sources. The goal is to provide balanced nutrition while ensuring that foods are easily digestible.

Soft Food Diet:
The soft food diet introduces more texture and variety, including:

Weeks 5-6: Foods like scrambled eggs, soft cheeses, cooked grains, and tender meats or fish. The emphasis is on maintaining a balanced diet while adapting to a broader range of textures.

Transition to Solid Foods:

As you progress in your recovery, you will gradually reintroduce solid foods. This typically occurs around the 6 to 8-week mark. However, the timing may vary based on your surgeon's recommendations and your individual progress.

Nutritional Considerations:

Maintaining proper nutrition is vital during your post-operative journey. Here are some key considerations:

- **Protein Intake:** Protein is essential for wound healing and preserving lean body mass. You should aim to meet your daily protein requirements as recommended by your dietitian.

- **Hydration:** Staying well-hydrated is crucial. Sip water throughout the day and avoid drinking with meals to prevent overeating.

- **Supplementation:** Depending on the type of weight loss surgery you've had, you may require nutritional supplements to prevent deficiencies. Common supplements include multivitamins, calcium, vitamin D, and vitamin B12.

- **Portion Control:** Be mindful of portion sizes. Overeating can lead to discomfort and may hinder your weight loss progress.

- **Fiber and Vegetables:** As you transition to solid foods, gradually incorporate fiber-rich foods and vegetables into your diet to support digestive health.

Long-Term Nutrition:

Weight loss surgery necessitates a lifelong commitment to nutritional wellness. After the initial recovery period, your dietitian will continue to provide guidance on meal planning, portion control, and nutrient-rich choices. It's essential to:

- Maintain regular follow-up appointments with your dietitian and surgical team.
- Pay attention to your body's cues for hunger and fullness.
- Be mindful of the types of foods you consume, focusing on quality nutrition.

Emotional and Behavioral Eating:

Weight loss surgery often addresses physical aspects of overeating, but it's crucial to address emotional and behavioral factors that contribute to unhealthy eating habits. Seek support from a therapist or counselor if you encounter emotional challenges during your journey.

Self-Image and Body Positivity:

Your body will undergo significant changes, and it's important to embrace a positive self-image and practice self-compassion. Develop a healthy self-concept and acknowledge your progress along the way.

Exercise and Physical Activity in Weight Loss Surgery

Exercise and physical activity are integral components of a successful weight loss surgery journey. Let's discuss the importance of exercise, the types of activities you can engage in, and how to establish a fitness routine that complements your post-operative lifestyle.

1. The Importance of Exercise:

Exercise offers numerous benefits in the context of weight loss surgery, including:

Weight Management: Regular physical activity contributes to weight loss and helps maintain a healthy weight.

Muscle Preservation: Exercise helps preserve lean body mass, ensuring that you lose primarily fat rather than muscle.

Metabolism Boost: Physical activity increases your metabolism, aiding in calorie expenditure.

Cardiovascular Health: Exercise improves heart and lung health, reducing the risk of cardiovascular diseases.

Mood Enhancement: Regular exercise can boost mood, reduce stress, and enhance overall well-being.

Enhanced Mobility: Improved physical fitness and strength enhance your ability to perform daily activities.

2. Types of Exercise:

Various types of exercise can be part of your post-operative fitness routine. Consider incorporating the following:

Cardiovascular Exercise: Activities like walking, swimming, cycling, or aerobic classes help improve cardiovascular fitness and burn calories.

Strength Training: Strength training with weights or resistance bands builds and maintains muscle mass.

Flexibility and Stretching: Stretching exercises enhance flexibility and reduce the risk of injury.

Balance and Core Work: Exercises that target balance and core strength can improve stability and posture.

Functional Training: Functional exercises mimic everyday movements, improving overall functional fitness.

3. Establishing a Fitness Routine:

Creating a fitness routine that suits your post-operative lifestyle is essential. Here's how to get started:

Consult Your Healthcare Team: Before beginning any exercise program, consult your surgeon or healthcare team to ensure that you are cleared for physical activity. They can provide personalized recommendations based on your specific surgery and recovery progress.

Start Slowly: If you're new to exercise, start with low-impact activities. Increase duration and intensity gradually over time.

Establish Achievable Fitness Objectives That Match Your Current Physical Capabilities: Set realistic fitness objectives. Appreciating little accomplishments along the road is crucial.

The Secret Is Consistency: Consistency is more crucial than intensity.

Aim for regular, sustainable exercise rather than sporadic, high-intensity workouts.

Enjoyment Matters: Choose activities you enjoy. You're more likely to stick with an exercise routine if you find it fun and engaging.

Work with a Professional: Consider working with a certified personal trainer or physical therapist who specializes in post-bariatric exercise to receive tailored guidance and support.

Safety First: Listen to your body. If you experience pain or discomfort during exercise, stop and consult your healthcare team. Hydration is also crucial, so drink water before, during, and after your workouts.

Mindful Eating: Exercise complements a healthy diet. Continue to focus on dietary modifications as you engage in physical activity.

4. Progress and Adjustments:

Your exercise routine may need adjustments as your body adapts and your fitness level improves. It's important to:

- Continually challenge yourself by increasing the intensity and variety of your workouts.

- Track your progress, which can be motivating and help you set new goals.

- Be mindful of any physical limitations, and communicate with your healthcare team as needed.

5. Emotional and Mental Well-Being:

Exercise not only benefits your physical health but also contributes to emotional and mental well-being. Frequent exercise can enhance mood, lower stress levels, and increase self-confidence. As you navigate the emotional aspects of your weight loss journey, exercise can be a valuable tool in maintaining a positive mindset.

6. Lifestyle Integration:

Ultimately, the goal is to integrate physical activity into your post-operative lifestyle in a sustainable way. Regular exercise contributes to long-term success in maintaining a healthier weight and overall well-being.

Emotional and Psychological Aspects of Weight Loss Surgery

Weight loss surgery is not only a physical transformation but also a profound emotional and psychological journey. This chapter delves into the emotional and psychological aspects of your weight loss surgery experience, addressing common challenges and offering guidance for a successful transition.

Pre-Operative Emotions:

Before undergoing weight loss surgery, it's common to experience a range of emotions, including:

- **Excitement:** Anticipation about the positive changes and improved health that surgery can bring.

- **Anxiety:** Concerns about the surgery itself, potential complications, or the recovery process.

- **Hope:** A sense of hope for a healthier and more fulfilling future.

- **Fear:** Apprehension about the unknown and the potential impact of the surgery on your life.

Post-Operative Emotional Challenges:

The post-operative phase often brings its own set of emotional challenges:

- **Body Image:** As your body undergoes rapid changes, you may experience shifts in body image. Some individuals struggle with excess skin or perceived imperfections, while others embrace their new bodies.

- **Social and Family Dynamics:** Your relationships with friends and family may evolve. Some people may feel jealousy or discomfort as you experience positive changes, while others provide unwavering support.

- **Emotional Eating:** Emotional eating is a common challenge. Surgery can address physical aspects of overeating, but emotional and psychological factors may persist. See a therapist or counselor for assistance in controlling your emotional eating.

- **Mental Health:** Mental health considerations are vital. Some individuals may face post-operative depression, anxiety, or adjustment difficulties.

Professional support is available to address these concerns.

Behavioral Changes:

Successful weight loss surgery involves adopting and maintaining healthy behavioral changes. These include:

- **Dietary Modifications:** Adhering to dietary guidelines and portion control.

- **Physical Activity:** Establishing and maintaining a regular exercise routine.

- **Stress management:** It is the process of creating constructive coping mechanisms to avoid emotional eating.

Support System:

A strong support system is invaluable during your weight loss surgery journey. Seek the support of friends, family, and peers who understand your experience. Participating in online forums or support groups can offer insightful conversations as well as emotional support.

Professional Counseling:

Professional counseling can be immensely beneficial in addressing emotional and psychological aspects:

- **Therapists or Counselors:** Therapists who specialize in bariatric care can help you navigate emotional challenges and behavioral changes.

Psychological Assessments: Some individuals may benefit from psychological assessments to identify underlying factors that contribute to overeating or other challenges.

Self-Compassion and Mindfulness:

Practice self-compassion and mindfulness as you navigate the emotional and psychological aspects of your journey:

- **Self-Compassion:** Be kind and forgiving toward yourself. Acknowledge that setbacks may occur and that it's okay to seek help when needed.

- **Mindfulness:** Develop mindfulness practices to stay present and aware of your emotions, thoughts, and behaviors. This can help you make conscious, healthy choices.

Setting Realistic Expectations:

Weight loss surgery is a tool for weight management and health improvement, but it is not a magic solution. Set realistic expectations for your journey and remember that it involves work, commitment, and time.

Post-Operative Adjustment:

The post-operative adjustment period varies for each individual. Give yourself time to adapt to your new body and lifestyle. Celebrate your successes and acknowledge your resilience in the face of challenges.

Seeking Help When Needed:

If you encounter emotional or psychological difficulties that hinder your progress, don't hesitate to seek professional help. Mental health support is a valuable resource in your journey.

Mindful Eating:

By connecting with your body's signals of hunger and fullness, mindful eating can help you prevent overindulging and emotional eating.

Long-Term Outcomes and Complications in Weight Loss Surgery

Long-term outcomes and potential complications are critical considerations in the journey of weight loss surgery. This chapter provides insights into what you can expect in the years following your surgery, as well as an understanding of potential complications and how to mitigate them.

Long-Term Weight Loss and Health Outcomes:

Weight loss surgery can lead to significant long-term health improvements, including:

- **Sustained Weight Loss:** Many individuals experience substantial and sustained weight loss after surgery. Over time, this can result in a healthier body weight and reduced risk of obesity-related health issues.

- Improvements in Co-Morbidities: Conditions like type 2 diabetes, hypertension, sleep apnea, and joint pain often improve or resolve after surgery.

- **Enhanced Quality of Life:** Weight loss surgery can lead to an improved quality of life, including increased mobility, self-confidence, and overall well-being.

- **Increased Longevity:** By reducing the risk of obesity-related health problems, surgery may contribute to a longer, healthier life.

Potential Long-Term Complications:

While weight loss surgery offers numerous benefits, potential complications can arise. It's essential to be aware of these and take proactive measures to mitigate them:

- **Nutritional Deficiencies**: Malabsorption or reduced food intake may lead to nutritional deficiencies. Regular follow-up with a dietitian and adherence to supplementation guidelines can help prevent deficiencies.

- **Excess Skin:** After significant weight loss, some individuals may experience excess skin. This can be addressed through plastic surgery procedures if desired.

- **Gallstones:** Losing weight quickly can make gallstones more likely. Your healthcare team can offer guidance on preventing and managing this complication.

- **Dumping Syndrome:** Some individuals may experience dumping syndrome, characterized by nausea, vomiting, and diarrhea after consuming certain foods high in sugar or fat. Adhering to dietary guidelines can help avoid this issue.

- **Vitamin and Mineral Deficiencies:** Specific vitamin and mineral deficiencies, such as vitamin B12, iron, and calcium, may occur. Regular blood tests and supplementation are essential for prevention.

Lifelong Follow-Up and Monitoring:

Lifelong follow-up and monitoring with your healthcare team are crucial to address and prevent potential complications:

Regular Medical Check-Ups: Schedule regular check-ups with your surgeon and primary care physician to monitor your overall health.

Nutritional Evaluation: Continue to work with a dietitian to assess and address nutritional needs.

Vitamin and Mineral Supplementation: Adhere to recommended vitamin and mineral supplementation to prevent deficiencies.

Behavioral Support: If you experience emotional or psychological challenges related to your journey, seek support from a therapist or counselor.

Long-Term Success and Lifestyle Maintenance:

Long-term success in weight loss surgery depends on the maintenance of healthy lifestyle habits:

- **Diet:** Continue to follow a balanced, nutrient-dense diet and portion control. Avoid reverting to previous eating habits.

- **Exercise:** Maintain a regular exercise routine to support weight maintenance and overall health.

- **Emotional and Behavioral Health**: Take care of any psychological issues and emotional eating that might be influencing your path.

- **Support System:** Maintain a strong support system through family, friends, support groups, and healthcare professionals.

- **Mindfulness**: Practice mindfulness and self-compassion to stay aware of your body's needs and maintain a positive self-image.

Revision Surgery:

In some cases, individuals may require revision surgery due to complications, insufficient weight loss, or weight regain. Your healthcare team can evaluate your individual circumstances and determine if revision surgery is appropriate.

Staying Informed:

Staying informed about the latest research and developments in bariatric care is valuable. New treatments, procedures, and guidelines may emerge over time.

Your Unique Journey:

Remember that your weight loss surgery journey is unique. While there are general trends and expectations, individual experiences and outcomes can vary. Regular communication with your healthcare team and a proactive approach to addressing any challenges that arise will contribute to your long-term success.

Long-Term Benefits of Gastric Sleeve Surgery:

Gastric sleeve surgery, also known as sleeve gastrectomy, offers a range of long-term benefits for individuals struggling with obesity and its related health issues. These benefits include:

Significant and Sustainable Weight Loss: Gastric sleeve surgery leads to substantial weight loss, and most individuals can maintain a healthier weight over the long term. The procedure removes a significant portion of the stomach, reducing its capacity and thus limiting food intake.

Resolution of Comorbidities: Many obesity-related co-morbidities, such as type 2 diabetes, high blood pressure, sleep apnea, and joint pain, often improve or resolve after gastric sleeve surgery. This improvement can lead to a better quality of life and reduced reliance on medications.

Improved Quality of Life: Weight loss and the resolution of health issues can lead to increased mobility, self-confidence, and an enhanced overall quality of life. Patients often report feeling more energetic and engaged in activities they couldn't participate in before surgery.

Reduced Risk of Cardiovascular Disease: By addressing obesity and related conditions, gastric sleeve surgery lowers the risk of cardiovascular diseases, including heart disease and stroke.

Enhanced Longevity: The combination of weight loss and improved health outcomes can contribute to a longer, healthier life, reducing the risk of premature mortality.

Fewer Restrictions on Food Choices: Unlike some other weight loss surgeries, such as gastric bypass, gastric sleeve surgery allows patients to eat a wide variety of foods in smaller quantities. This flexibility can enhance long-term adherence to a healthy diet.

Long-Term Benefits of Gastric Bypass Surgery:

Gastric bypass surgery, specifically the Roux-en-Y procedure, offers several long-term benefits for individuals seeking to address obesity and related health conditions. These benefits include:

Significant Weight Loss: Gastric bypass leads to substantial and sustained weight loss. It achieves this by restricting food intake and altering the way the body absorbs and processes nutrients.

Resolution of Comorbidities: Obesity-related co-morbidities, including type 2 diabetes, hypertension, and sleep apnea, often improve or resolve after gastric bypass surgery. Patients may experience reduced reliance on medications.

Improved Quality of Life: Weight loss and the resolution of health issues lead to increased mobility, self-esteem, and overall well-being. Patients often report greater enjoyment of life and a higher level of physical activity.

Lower Risk of Cardiovascular Disease: Gastric bypass can reduce the risk of cardiovascular diseases, such as heart disease and stroke, by addressing obesity and its associated risk factors.

Enhanced Longevity: Improved health outcomes and a reduction in obesity-related risks can contribute to a longer, healthier life, lowering the risk of premature mortality.

Effective Portion Control: Gastric bypass provides effective portion control by limiting the amount of food the stomach can hold. This helps patients maintain a healthier weight over the long term.

Reduced Caloric Absorption: By rerouting the digestive system, gastric bypass reduces the absorption of calories and nutrients from food, aiding in weight loss and long-term weight management.

Common Complications and Their Management in Weight Loss Surgery

Weight loss surgery, like any surgical procedure, can be associated with certain complications. While these complications are relatively rare, it's crucial to be aware of them and understand how they can be managed. Here, we will discuss some common complications and the ways they can be addressed.

1. Infection:

Common Complication: Surgical site infections can occur after weight loss surgery.

Management:

Prevention: Surgical teams follow strict infection control protocols during surgery to minimize the risk.

Treatment: If an infection occurs, it is typically treated with antibiotics. In some cases, drainage of an abscess may be required.

2. Leaks:

Common Complication: Leaks, which are small openings in the surgical connections, can happen.

Management:

Prevention: Surgeons take great care to create secure connections during the procedure.

Treatment: If a leak is suspected, it may require further surgery or placement of drains to resolve the issue. Early detection is crucial to prevent complications.

3. Bleeding:

Common Complication: Post-operative bleeding can occur, leading to symptoms like pain, swelling, or low blood pressure.

Management:

Prevention: Surgeons employ meticulous techniques to minimize the risk of bleeding during surgery.

Treatment: If bleeding occurs, it may be managed with blood transfusions, endoscopy, or, in rare cases, re-operation.

4. Nutritional Deficiencies:

Common Complication: Nutritional deficiencies can develop over time, particularly in surgeries with malabsorptive elements like gastric bypass.

Management:

Prevention: Regular follow-up with a dietitian and adherence to nutritional guidelines.
Treatment: Nutritional deficiencies are managed through supplements and dietary adjustments. Some individuals may require lifelong supplementation.

5. Dumping Syndrome:

Common Complication: Dumping syndrome can occur in surgeries that involve rerouting the digestive system, like gastric bypass. It leads to symptoms like nausea, vomiting, and diarrhea after consuming certain foods.

Management:

Prevention: Avoiding high-sugar and high-fat foods can prevent dumping syndrome.

Treatment: Dietary adjustments can alleviate symptoms. Medication may be prescribed under certain circumstances.

6. Ulcers:

Common Complication: Ulcers may form in the stomach or small intestine following weight loss surgery.

Management:

Prevention: Avoiding smoking and non-steroidal anti-inflammatory drugs (NSAIDs) can reduce the risk.

Treatment: Medications and lifestyle changes can manage ulcers. Endoscopic operations might be necessary in extreme situations.

7. Gallstones:

Common Complication: Rapid weight loss can increase the risk of gallstones.

Management:
Prevention: Some surgeons recommend removing the gallbladder during weight loss surgery to prevent gallstones.

Treatment: If gallstones occur, they may require removal through surgery or nonsurgical methods.

8. Excess Skin:

Common Complication: After significant weight loss, excess skin may remain.

Management:

Prevention: Maintaining hydration and muscle mass during weight loss can minimize excess skin.

Treatment: Cosmetic surgery procedures can remove excess skin if desired.

9. Emotional and Psychological Challenges:

Common Complication: Emotional and psychological challenges, such as depression, anxiety, or emotional eating, can affect some individuals.

Management:

Prevention: Engaging in counseling and support groups can help prevent or address these challenges.

Treatment: Therapists or counselors can provide support and guidance for managing emotional and psychological aspects.

10. Revision Surgery:

Common Complication: Some individuals may require revision surgery due to complications, insufficient weight loss, or weight regain.

Management:

Assessment: Your healthcare team will assess your individual circumstances and determine if revision surgery is necessary.

Success Stories and Challenges in Weight Loss Surgery

Weight loss surgery is a transformative journey that often comes with inspiring success stories and unique challenges. Let's explore both the successes and the obstacles that individuals may encounter during and after their weight loss surgery experience.

Success Stories:

Remarkable Weight Loss: Many individuals achieve remarkable weight loss success after surgery, shedding a substantial amount of excess weight. These success stories often come with improved health and increased mobility.

Resolution of Comorbidities: Weight loss surgery frequently leads to the resolution of obesity-related co-morbidities, such as type 2 diabetes, hypertension, sleep apnea, and joint pain. Patients report reduced reliance on medications and a better quality of life.

Enhanced Quality of Life: Success stories include an enhanced quality of life, with individuals experiencing increased energy, self-confidence, and an ability to engage in activities they couldn't participate in before surgery.

Positive Body Image: Many patients develop a positive body image as they embrace their transformed appearance and new-found health. They celebrate their post-surgery bodies and the journey they've undertaken.

Inspiration for Others: Weight loss surgery success stories often inspire and motivate others to consider and embark on their own weight loss journey. Sharing personal experiences can empower individuals to make positive changes in their lives.

Challenges:

Physical and Emotional Challenges: Weight loss surgery may involve physical challenges during recovery, including pain and discomfort. Overcoming emotional obstacles can also include handling emotional eating and adjusting to a new body image.

Lifestyle Adjustments: Adapting to the necessary lifestyle changes can be challenging, including dietary modifications, regular exercise, and the need for ongoing medical and nutritional follow-up.

Support and Social Dynamics: Some individuals may encounter challenges in their support systems and social dynamics. Friends and family may react differently to the changes, which can lead to feelings of isolation or tension.

Plateaus and Regain: Weight loss is not always linear, and individuals may experience plateaus or regain some weight. These periods can be discouraging but are common in the weight loss journey.

Nutritional Deficiencies: The risk of nutritional deficiencies is an ongoing challenge, particularly in surgeries with malabsorptive elements. Regular follow-up with a dietitian and adherence to supplementation guidelines are necessary.

Dumping Syndrome: For those who undergo procedures like gastric bypass, dumping syndrome can be a challenge. Managing the symptoms and avoiding triggering foods can be difficult.

Emotional and Psychological Factors: Addressing emotional and psychological factors that contribute to overeating or emotional eating is an ongoing challenge for some individuals. Getting help from counselors or therapists is crucial.

Revisions and Complications: In some cases, individuals may require revision surgery due to complications or unsatisfactory outcomes. These circumstances can be taxing on the body and the emotions.

Balancing Success and Challenges:

Successful weight loss surgery journeys involve a balance of celebrating achievements and facing challenges. Overcoming obstacles and persisting through difficult times are integral to the long-term success of weight loss surgery. Having a strong support system, regular follow-up with healthcare professionals, and a proactive approach to addressing challenges can help individuals navigate their unique weight loss journey.

Every Journey Is Unique:

It's important to remember that every weight loss surgery journey is unique, and individual experiences vary. Celebrating the successes and embracing the challenges are part of what makes each story distinctive and inspiring. By sharing experiences and offering support to others, those who have undergone weight loss surgery can encourage and guide individuals who are considering or embarking on their own journey to better health and well-being.

Real-Life Insights into Weight Loss Surgery

Gaining real-life insights into weight loss surgery from individuals who have experienced the journey can provide valuable guidance and inspiration. In this chapter, we explore personal stories and lessons from those who have undergone weight loss surgery.

Personal Transformations:

Weight loss surgery often marks the beginning of a personal transformation. Individuals share how their lives changed, not just physically, but emotionally and mentally. They recount stories of newfound confidence, improved self-esteem, and a rekindled sense of self-worth.

Coping with Emotional Eating:

Many share their experiences of coping with emotional eating. They reveal strategies for managing the emotional aspects of overeating and finding healthier ways to deal with stress, anxiety, and sadness. Support from therapists and counselors is often instrumental in this process.

Relationship Dynamics:

Navigating changes in relationships with family, friends, and partners is a common theme. Some share stories of unwavering support and understanding, while others discuss challenges in dealing with jealousy or discomfort as their appearance and lifestyle transform.

Staying Committed to Health:

Real-life insights often emphasize the importance of staying committed to health and well-being. Individuals talk about adhering to dietary and exercise guidelines and making conscious choices to maintain their weight loss and health improvements.

Realistic Expectations:

Many who have undergone weight loss surgery stress the significance of setting realistic expectations. They encourage individuals to remember that surgery is a tool and not a magic solution, and that the journey may involve setbacks and plateaus.

Celebrating Milestones:

Individuals celebrate personal milestones and achievements, whether it's fitting into smaller-sized clothing, participating in physical activities they couldn't before, or reaching significant weight loss goals. These stories serve as reminders of the rewards that come with dedication and perseverance.

Ongoing Support:

Real-life insights underscore the value of ongoing support from healthcare teams, dietitians, and therapists. Individuals stress the importance of attending regular follow-up appointments and seeking help when needed, whether for emotional or physical challenges.

Managing Nutritional Needs:

Many share insights into managing nutritional needs. They discuss the importance of a balanced diet and supplementation, especially in surgeries with malabsorptive elements. Staying mindful of nutritional requirements is vital for long-term success.

Addressing Complications:

Individuals who have faced complications or needed revision surgery stress the importance of early detection and proactive management. Sharing their experiences can offer guidance to others who may encounter similar challenges.

Body Positivity:

Real-life insights often emphasize the significance of body positivity and self-acceptance. Stories of embracing post-surgery bodies and the scars that come with it can inspire self-love and a healthy self-image.

Aftercare and Support in Weight Loss Surgery

After undergoing weight loss surgery, ongoing aftercare and support play a vital role in ensuring long-term success and maintaining a healthier weight and lifestyle. This chapter explores the importance of aftercare and the types of support available to individuals who have undergone weight loss surgery.

The Importance of Ongoing Medical Follow-ups in Weight Loss Surgery

After weight loss surgery, ongoing medical follow-ups are not just recommended; they are essential for the long-term health and well-being of individuals who have undergone these procedures. The critical importance of regular post-operative medical check-ups is as follows:

Health Monitoring:

Ongoing medical follow-ups serve as a fundamental means of monitoring your overall health. Post-surgery appointments allow healthcare professionals to assess your progress, detect potential complications early, and ensure that you are on track with your weight loss and health goals.

Early Detection of Complications:

One of the primary purposes of medical follow-ups is the early detection of complications. While complications are relatively rare in weight loss surgery, they can occur, and their prompt identification is crucial for effective management and resolution.

Nutritional and Supplement Assessment:

Medical follow-ups include assessments of nutritional status and supplementation needs. Weight loss surgery can affect nutrient absorption, so regular evaluations are essential to detect and prevent nutritional deficiencies.

Medication Adjustments:

Weight loss surgery can alter the way medications are absorbed and metabolized in the body. Medical follow-ups are necessary to assess and adjust medication regimens as needed.

Behavioral and Emotional Health:

Medical follow-ups often include evaluations of emotional and psychological well-being. Addressing emotional and psychological factors that contribute to overeating or other challenges is integral to long-term success.

Weight and Health Progress:

Follow-up appointments provide an opportunity to assess your weight loss progress and overall health. Your healthcare team can guide you on whether further adjustments are needed in your dietary or lifestyle choices.

Support and Guidance:

Medical follow-ups offer a support system. Your healthcare team can provide guidance, answer your questions, and offer reassurance during moments of uncertainty. This ongoing support is essential for maintaining motivation and adherence to post-surgery recommendations.

Advocating for Your Health:

In post-surgery medical follow-ups, it's essential to advocate for your health. Don't hesitate to ask questions, express concerns, and seek clarification on any aspects of your post-surgery journey.

Regularity of Appointments:

The frequency of follow-up appointments may vary based on individual circumstances and the specific surgery performed. In the early post-operative period, appointments are often more frequent and gradually become less frequent as time goes on. Adherence to the recommended schedule is crucial for long-term success.

Long-Term Well-Being:

The overarching goal of medical follow-ups is to support your long-term well-being. By attending these appointments and maintaining open communication with your healthcare team, you can mitigate potential complications, ensure proper nutrition and supplementation management, and work towards a healthier and more fulfilling life after weight loss surgery.

Support Groups and Resources in the Weight Loss Surgery Journey

Weight loss surgery is a transformative journey that benefits greatly from a strong support system and access to valuable resources. In this chapter, we explore the importance of support groups and the wealth of resources available to individuals who have undergone or are considering weight loss surgery.

The Power of Support Groups:

Support groups are gatherings of individuals who share common experiences and challenges. In the context of weight loss surgery, support groups offer a unique and invaluable source of assistance and inspiration.

Key Benefits of Support Groups:

Emotional Support: Body image, self-esteem, and emotional eating are just a few of the psychological and emotional issues that support groups offer as a safe place to talk about in relation to weight reduction surgery.

Shared Experiences: Individuals who have undergone weight loss surgery can relate to each other's experiences, providing a sense of camaraderie and understanding.

Practical Insights: Support group members often share practical insights, tips, and strategies that have worked for them in managing the post-surgery journey.

Accountability: Regular meetings can help individuals stay accountable for their dietary and lifestyle choices, motivating them to adhere to recommendations.

Motivation and Inspiration: Hearing the success stories and accomplishments of others can be highly motivating and inspiring.

Types of Support Groups:

Support groups come in various forms, including:

In-Person Groups: These are local gatherings where individuals meet face-to-face to share their experiences.

Online Communities: Virtual communities and forums provide a platform for individuals to connect, share their journeys, and seek advice from a wider audience.

Hospital-Based Groups: Many hospitals and medical centers offer post-surgery support groups as part of their comprehensive care programs.

Patient Advocacy Organizations: Numerous patient advocacy organizations, such as the American Society for Metabolic and Bariatric Surgery (ASMBS), provide resources and support through in-person and online groups.

Resources for Weight Loss Surgery:

In addition to support groups, a wealth of resources is available to individuals who have undergone or are considering weight loss surgery:

Dietitians: Dietitians specializing in bariatric nutrition can provide personalized guidance on maintaining a balanced diet and proper supplementation.

Exercise Specialists: Exercise specialists can tailor fitness programs to align with an individual's physical abilities and weight loss goals.

Therapists and Counselors: Therapy and counseling services are available to address emotional and psychological challenges related to weight loss surgery, including depression, anxiety, and emotional eating.

Nutritional and Weight Management Classes: Classes and seminars on nutrition, healthy cooking, and weight management are offered to help individuals make informed choices.

Body Image and Self-Esteem Workshops: Workshops focusing on body positivity and self-acceptance can be valuable in promoting a positive self-image.

Patient Advocacy Organizations: These organizations often provide educational materials, webinars, and patient resources to support individuals through their weight loss surgery journey.

Online Forums and Websites: Numerous websites, forums, and blogs share information, stories, and resources related to weight loss surgery. These may be very helpful resources for knowledge and ideas.

Balancing Support and Resources:

Effective navigation of the weight loss surgery journey involves balancing the support of a community with access to valuable resources. Support groups offer personal connections, emotional understanding, and motivation, while resources such as dietitians, therapists, and classes provide professional guidance and education.

Advocating for Your Needs:

When seeking support and resources, don't hesitate to advocate for your unique needs. Each individual's weight loss surgery journey is distinctive, and your requirements may vary. Be proactive in seeking the assistance and information that aligns with your specific circumstances.

Maintaining a Healthy Lifestyle After Weight Loss Surgery

Weight loss surgery is a significant step in your journey towards improved health and well-being. To ensure the long-term success of your surgery and maintain a healthy lifestyle, you'll need to make lasting changes to your diet, exercise routine, and overall mindset. In this chapter, we'll explore key principles for maintaining a healthy lifestyle after weight loss surgery.

Embrace a Balanced Diet:

After weight loss surgery, your stomach's capacity to hold food is significantly reduced. To maintain a healthy lifestyle, it's essential to focus on a balanced diet:

- **Protein Priority:** Prioritize protein-rich foods to support muscle health and promote satiety.

-

- **Limit Sugars and Refined Carbs:** Sugary and highly processed foods can lead to dumping syndrome and hinder weight loss. Avoid them as much as possible.

-

- **Portion Control:** Be mindful of serving sizes and refrain from overindulging. A smaller stomach means smaller meals.

-

- **Stay Hydrated:** Drink plenty of water throughout the day to prevent dehydration and promote overall health.

-

- **Fruits and Vegetables:** Incorporate a variety of fruits and vegetables into your diet to ensure a range of nutrients.

- **Fiber Intake:** Choose high-fiber foods to support digestive health and aid in feeling full.

Regular Exercise:

Exercise is essential to keeping up a healthy lifestyle. Regular physical activity helps with weight management, increases energy levels, and promotes overall well-being. Aim for a combination of aerobic exercises, strength training, and flexibility exercises that suit your physical abilities and preferences.

Vitamins and Supplements:

Weight loss surgery can lead to nutritional deficiencies, so it's important to follow your healthcare team's recommendations for vitamins and supplements. These may include vitamin

B12, vitamin D, calcium, and iron, among others.

Emotional and Psychological Well-Being:

Addressing emotional and psychological aspects is a significant part of maintaining a healthy lifestyle:

- **Therapy & Counseling:** To deal with emotional difficulties including sadness, anxiety, and emotional eating, get expert assistance.

- **Mindful Eating:** Pay attention to hunger and fullness cues, and avoid emotional eating or eating out of habit.

- **Positive Self-Image:** Cultivate a positive body image and self-esteem. Focus on the progress you've made and embrace your transformed self.

Support and Follow-Up:

Regular follow-up appointments with your healthcare team are vital for monitoring your progress, addressing potential complications, and making necessary adjustments to your diet and lifestyle. Support groups and online communities provide a sense of camaraderie and motivation in your journey.

Setting Realistic Goals:

Setting achievable, realistic goals is crucial for maintaining a healthy lifestyle. Focus on making gradual, sustainable changes rather than aiming for rapid results. Celebrate your achievements, whether they are related to weight loss, fitness, or overall well-being.

Balance and Flexibility:

Maintaining a healthy lifestyle is about balance and flexibility. While adhering to dietary and exercise guidelines is important, it's also essential to allow yourself occasional treats and moments of relaxation. Life is about enjoyment as well.

Stay Informed:

Stay informed about the latest developments in weight loss surgery and related treatments. Knowledge is a valuable tool in making informed choices about your health and well-being.

Taking Control of Your Health After Weight Loss Surgery

Weight loss surgery is a pivotal moment in your journey towards better health and well-being, but the real transformative power lies in the choices you make and your commitment to taking control of your health. In this chapter, we will explore the key steps to help you maintain your health and maximize the benefits of weight loss surgery.

Empowering Knowledge:

One of the first steps in taking control of your health is to become informed. Understand the specifics of your weight loss surgery, its potential risks and benefits, and the lifestyle changes that will be necessary for success. You can make more informed decisions regarding your health when you are well-informed.

Commitment to Lifestyle Changes:

Weight loss surgery is a tool, not a magic solution. Your long-term success depends on your commitment to making and maintaining lifestyle changes. This includes a balanced diet, regular exercise, and emotional well-being. Strive for consistency and patience as you adapt to these changes.

Regular Medical Follow-ups:

Regular medical follow-ups are vital for monitoring your progress, detecting potential complications, and ensuring that you are on track with your weight loss and health goals. Attend these appointments diligently and communicate openly with your healthcare team.

Balanced Diet:

Embrace a balanced diet that prioritizes protein, minimizes sugars and refined carbs, practices portion control, and includes a variety of fruits and vegetables. A dietitian can provide personalized guidance to meet your nutritional needs.

Regular Exercise:

Regular physical activity is crucial for maintaining your health. Engage in a combination of aerobic exercises, strength training, and flexibility exercises that align with your abilities and preferences.

Emotional and Psychological Well-being:

Your mental health is an integral part of your overall well-being. Seek therapy or counseling if you encounter emotional challenges related to body image, self-esteem, or emotional eating. Cultivate a positive self-image and embrace your transformed self.

Support and Resources:

Lean on the support of support groups, online communities, and valuable resources that provide insights, camaraderie, and motivation. Utilize dietitians, therapists, and other professionals to guide you through your journey.

Setting Realistic Goals:

Set achievable, realistic goals and celebrate your achievements, whether they are related to weight loss, fitness, or overall well-being. Prioritize sustainable, slow growth over quick fixes.

Advocating for Your Needs:

Advocate for your unique needs and communicate openly with your healthcare team. Each weight loss surgery journey is unique, and your requirements may differ from others.

Staying Informed:

Stay informed about the latest developments in weight loss surgery and related treatments. You may make decisions regarding your health and well-being that are more informed when you have knowledge.

Positive Mindset:

A positive mindset is a powerful tool in taking control of your health. Focus on the progress you've made, embrace self-acceptance, and cultivate a sense of gratitude for your healthier, happier life.

Balance and Flexibility:

Maintaining your health is about balance and flexibility. While adhering to dietary and exercise guidelines is important, it's also essential to allow yourself occasional treats and moments of relaxation. A healthy life includes enjoyment.

Conclusion

Empowering Your Weight Loss Surgery Journey:

In the course of this book, we have embarked on a transformative journey, exploring the multifaceted world of weight loss surgery. From the initial considerations to the post-operative steps and lifelong commitments, this journey is one of self-discovery, health transformation, and empowerment. As we conclude, let's reflect on the key takeaways and the overarching message that this journey imparts.

Weight loss surgery is a remarkable tool for achieving improved health, physical well-being, and an enhanced quality of life. It's a journey that begins with careful consideration, thorough preparation, and a clear understanding of the procedures, potential outcomes, and the changes it will entail. Armed with this knowledge, individuals embark on a path that demands unwavering commitment to lifestyle adjustments, a balanced diet, regular exercise, and emotional well-being.

Throughout this journey, we've emphasized the importance of setting realistic goals and maintaining a positive mindset. Weight loss surgery is a transformative process, but it is not a magic solution. Success comes from dedication, patience, and the resilience to overcome challenges and setbacks. Each step forward, no matter how small, brings you closer to your health and wellness goals.

Support, both from your healthcare team and support groups, is an invaluable resource on this journey. Regular follow-up appointments, dietary guidance, and emotional support help keep you on track. Additionally, connecting with individuals who share similar experiences creates a sense of camaraderie, understanding, and motivation.

Your commitment to lifestyle changes is a testament to your desire for a healthier, happier life. Maintaining a balanced diet, regular exercise, and emotional well-being is a lifelong endeavor. It's about embracing change, seeking out knowledge, and advocating for your unique needs. The power to take control of your health lies within you, and your journey is a testament to your strength and determination.

As we conclude this book, we celebrate the empowerment that weight loss surgery offers. It is not just a journey of physical transformation; it is a voyage of self-discovery, resilience, and personal growth. Every individual's experience is unique, and your success is defined by your dedication and the choices you make on this path.

In your pursuit of a healthier, happier life, always remember that your journey is a testament to your strength, resilience, and commitment to self-improvement. By embracing the changes and challenges that come your way, you are not just transforming your body; you are embracing the power to transform your life. Your future is filled with potential, and your health and well-being are now in your capable hands.

So, as you move forward on your weight loss surgery journey, we encourage you to continue embracing change, advocating for your needs, and celebrating the remarkable transformation you've achieved. You are the author of your health story, and the pages ahead are waiting for you to write them with determination, courage, and the knowledge that you have the power to live your best, healthiest life.

Appendix

10 sample meal plans along with corresponding recipes:

 to help you maintain a balanced and nutritious diet after weight loss surgery:

Sample Meal Plan 1: Protein-Packed Breakfast

Breakfast: Protein-Packed Omelet

Ingredients:
- 2 large eggs
- 1/4 cup diced bell peppers
- 1/4 cup diced onions
- 1/4 cup diced tomatoes
- 1/4 cup lean ground turkey
- Salt and pepper to taste

Instructions:
1. In a non-stick skillet, cook the lean ground turkey until browned.

2. Remove turkey from the skillet and set aside.

3. In the same skillet, sauté the bell peppers and onions until tender.

4. Beat the eggs, add them to the skillet, and scramble with the vegetables.

5. Mix in the cooked turkey and diced tomatoes.

6. Season with salt and pepper to taste.

Sample Meal Plan 2: Mediterranean Lunch

Lunch: Mediterranean Chickpea Salad

Ingredients:
- One cup of rinsed and drained canned chickpeas
- 1/4 cup diced cucumbers
- 1/4 cup diced tomatoes
- 2 tablespoons feta cheese
- 1 tablespoon olive oil
- 1 tablespoon lemon juice
- Fresh parsley for garnish

- Salt and pepper to taste

Instructions:
1. In a bowl, combine chickpeas, cucumbers, tomatoes, and feta cheese.
2. Drizzle with olive oil and lemon juice.
3. Season with salt and pepper.
4. Garnish with fresh parsley.

Sample Meal Plan 3: Snack Time

Snack: Cottage Cheese with Berries

Ingredients:
- 1/2 cup low-fat cottage cheese
- 1/4 cup of mixed berries, such as raspberries and blueberries

Instructions:
1. Combine cottage cheese with mixed berries for a creamy and satisfying snack.

Sample Meal Plan 4: Asian-Inspired Dinner

Dinner: Teriyaki Salmon with Broccoli and Brown Rice

Ingredients:
- 4 ounces salmon filet
- 1 cup steamed broccoli florets
- 1/2 cup cooked brown rice
- 2 tablespoons teriyaki sauce
- Garnish with green onions and sesame seeds.

Instructions:
1. Preheat your oven to 375°F (190°C).
2. Brush the salmon with teriyaki sauce.
3. Bake the salmon for about 15-20 minutes or until it's cooked through.
4. Serve with steamed broccoli and brown rice.
5. Add chopped green onions and sesame seeds as garnish.

Sample Meal Plan 5: Nut Butter Snack

Snack: Nut Butter and Apple Slices

Ingredients:
- 1 small apple, sliced
- 1 tablespoon nut butter (e.g., almond, peanut)

Instructions:
1. Dip apple slices in nut butter for a satisfying and crunchy snack.

Sample Meal Plan 6: Vegetarian Delight

Lunch: Quinoa and Black Bean Salad**

Ingredients:
- 1 cup cooked quinoa
-1/2 cup washed and drained canned black beans
- 1/4 cup diced bell peppers (various colors)
- 1/4 cup corn (canned or frozen)
- 2 tablespoons vinaigrette dressing (balsamic or your choice)
- Fresh cilantro for garnish
- Salt and pepper to taste

Instructions:
1. In a bowl, combine cooked quinoa, black beans, bell peppers, and corn.
2. Drizzle with vinaigrette dressing.
3. Season with salt and pepper.
4. Garnish with fresh cilantro.

Sample Meal Plan 7: Poultry Dinner

Dinner: Herb-Roasted Chicken with Steamed Asparagus and Quinoa

Ingredients:
- 4 ounces skinless chicken breast
- 1 cup steamed asparagus spears
- 1/2 cup cooked quinoa
- 1 tablespoon olive oil
- Fresh herbs (e.g., rosemary, thyme) for seasoning
- Salt and pepper to taste

Instructions:

1. Preheat your oven to 375°F (190°C).

2. Season the chicken breast with olive oil, fresh herbs, salt, and pepper.

3. Roast the chicken for about 25-30 minutes or until it's cooked through.

4. Serve with steamed asparagus and quinoa.

Sample Meal Plan 8: Afternoon Snack

Snack: Greek Yogurt Parfait

Ingredients:
- 1/2 cup Greek yogurt
- 1/4 cup granola
- 1/4 cup of mixed berries, such as blueberries and strawberries
- Honey for drizzling (optional)

Instructions:

1. Arrange mixed berries, granola, and Greek yogurt in a glass or bowl.

2. Drizzle honey over the top for extra sweetness.

Sample Meal Plan 9: Mexican Flavors

Lunch: Turkey and Black Bean Lettuce Wraps

Ingredients:
- 4 ounces lean ground turkey
- 1/2 cup canned black beans, washed and drained
- 1/4 cup diced tomatoes
- 1/4 cup diced red onions
- Romaine lettuce leaves for wrapping
- Salsa for garnish
- Fresh cilantro for garnish
- Salt and pepper to taste

Instructions:
1. In a skillet, cook the ground turkey until browned and season with salt and pepper.

2. In a bowl, combine black beans, diced tomatoes, and red onions.
3. Place a few spoonfuls of the turkey mixture into a lettuce leaf.
4. Top with the black bean mixture, salsa, and fresh cilantro.
5. Wrap and enjoy.

Sample Meal Plan 10: Sweet Tooth Satisfier

Snack: Yogurt and Banana Sundae

Ingredients:
- 1/2 cup low-fat vanilla yogurt
- 1/2 banana, sliced
- 1 tablespoon chopped nuts (e.g., almonds, walnuts)
- 1 tablespoon honey

Instructions:
1. In a bowl, layer low-fat vanilla yogurt, banana slices, and chopped nuts.
2. Drizzle honey over the top for a sweet treat.

Exercise Routines and Fitness Tips for Post-Weight Loss Surgery

Regular physical activity is a crucial component of a healthy lifestyle, especially after weight loss surgery. Exercise not only supports weight maintenance but also contributes to improved overall well-being. Before beginning any exercise routine, consult with your healthcare team to ensure that it aligns with your specific recovery and fitness goals. Here are exercise routines and fitness tips tailored for individuals post-weight loss surgery:

Start Slow and Gradual:
Begin with low-impact activities and gradually increase intensity. Walking is an excellent starting point, and as you build endurance, consider incorporating

other exercises like swimming, cycling, or low-impact aerobics.

Incorporate Strength Training:

Include strength training exercises to build and tone muscles. Major muscle areas including the arms, legs, and core should be your focus. Resistance bands or light weights can be used for added resistance.

Embrace Variety:

Diversify your exercise routine to keep things interesting and target different muscle groups. Mix cardiovascular exercises with strength training, flexibility exercises, and balance exercises.

Prioritize Posture and Form:

Maintain proper posture and form during exercises to prevent injuries. If unsure, consider working with a fitness professional, physical therapist, or attending classes that emphasize correct form.

Listen to Your Body:

Observe how your body reacts to physical activity. If you experience pain, discomfort, or fatigue, modify the intensity or duration of your workout. If you have any concerns, never hesitate to speak with your healthcare staff.

Set Realistic Goals:

Establish achievable fitness goals based on your current abilities. Celebrate small milestones and gradually increase the intensity and duration of your workouts as you become more comfortable with regular exercise.

Prioritize Cardiovascular Health:

Try to get in at least 150 minutes a week of aerobic activity at a moderate level. This can involve swimming, cycling, or brisk walking. Break it down into shorter sessions throughout the week for flexibility.

Flexibility and Stretching:
Incorporate stretches to increase range of motion and lower your chance of injury. Gentle stretching, yoga, or Pilates can be beneficial for enhancing flexibility and promoting relaxation.

Stay Hydrated:
Proper hydration is essential, especially during and after exercise. Carry a water bottle and drink water regularly throughout your workout to stay hydrated and support recovery.

Find Enjoyable Activities:
Choose exercises that you enjoy to make fitness a sustainable part of your routine. Whether it's dancing, hiking, or a group fitness class, finding activities you love increases the likelihood of consistency.

Schedule Regular Rest Days:
Allow your body time to rest and recover. Excessive training can cause weariness and possibly damage. Incorporate rest days into your weekly

routine to promote recovery and prevent burnout.

Consider Professional Guidance:
If you're unsure where to start or how to structure your exercise routine, consider working with a certified fitness professional or physical therapist. They can monitor your progress and customize a program to meet your unique needs.

Listen to Music or Podcasts:
Create a workout playlist or listen to engaging podcasts to make your exercise routine more enjoyable. Music and informative content can be motivating and distract you from the physical effort.

Involve a Workout Buddy:
Exercising with a friend or family member can add a social element to your routine, providing motivation and accountability. It can make the

experience more enjoyable and help you stay consistent.

Monitor Progress:
Keep track of your exercise routine and progress. Whether using a fitness app, journaling, or wearable fitness trackers, monitoring your achievements can boost motivation and highlight areas for improvement.

Glossary of Medical Terms for Weight Loss Surgery

Understanding the medical terminology associated with weight loss surgery is essential for effective communication with healthcare professionals and gaining insight into your own health. Here's a glossary of commonly used medical terms in the context of weight loss surgery:

A - D:

Adipose Tissue:

The scientific term for fat tissue, which stores energy in the form of fat.

Anastomosis:

A surgical connection between two structures. In weight loss surgery, it often refers to the connection between the stomach and the small intestine.

BMI (Body Mass Index):

A number determined by taking the height and weight of a person. It is commonly used to categorize individuals into weight status categories such as underweight, normal weight, overweight, and obesity.

Bariatric Surgery:

Operations on the intestines or stomach that are done to help people lose weight. Sleeve gastrectomy and gastric bypass are common varieties.

Dumping Syndrome:

A group of symptoms, including nausea and dizziness, that may occur after eating high-sugar or high-fat foods following certain types of weight loss surgery.

Dysphagia:

Difficulty swallowing, which may occur after weight loss surgery and usually improves over time.

E - H:

Endoscopy:

A medical procedure using a flexible tube with a light and camera to examine the interior of the digestive tract.

Gastric Bypass (Roux-en-Y):

A type of weight loss surgery that involves creating a small pouch from the stomach and connecting it directly to the small intestine, bypassing a portion of the stomach and the first part of the small intestine.

Gastric Sleeve (Sleeve Gastrectomy):

A weight loss surgery that involves removing a large portion of the stomach, leaving a sleeve-shaped tube.

Gastroenterologist:

A medical doctor who specializes in the diagnosis and treatment of disorders of the digestive system.

Hormone:

A chemical messenger produced by glands in the endocrine system that regulates various physiological functions, including metabolism and appetite.

I - P:

Intravenous (IV):

A method of delivering fluids or medications directly into a vein through a needle or catheter.

Laparoscopy:

A minimally invasive surgical technique using small incisions and a camera to view the inside of the body.

Nutrient Absorption:

The process by which nutrients from food are absorbed into the bloodstream through the walls of the gastrointestinal tract.

Obesity:

A medical condition characterized by an excess accumulation of body fat, often measured by a high BMI.

Port:

A small device implanted under the skin during weight loss surgery, allowing for the administration of medications or adjustments to certain procedures.

Q - Z:

Reflux:

The flow of stomach acid back into the esophagus, leading to symptoms such as heartburn.

Satiety:

The feeling of fullness or satisfaction after eating, influencing appetite and meal size.

Type 2 Diabetes:

A chronic condition characterized by elevated blood sugar levels, often associated with obesity. Weight loss surgery can lead to significant improvements or remission of type 2 diabetes.

Vitamin Deficiency:

Inadequate levels of essential vitamins in the body, which may occur after weight loss surgery due to changes in nutrient absorption.

Weight Loss Plateau:

A period during which an individual's weight remains stable despite ongoing efforts to lose weight.

Xerostomia:

Dry mouth, a condition that may be experienced after weight loss surgery.

Yoga:

A mind-body discipline that incorporates meditation, breath control, and physical postures. It can be a beneficial form of exercise after weight loss surgery.

Zinc:

An essential mineral involved in various bodily functions, including immune function and wound healing. Zinc deficiency may occur after weight loss surgery.

This glossary provides a starting point for understanding the medical terminology related to weight loss surgery. If you encounter unfamiliar terms, don't hesitate to consult with your healthcare team for clarification and guidance tailored to your specific situation.